What others are saying about

How Not to Be My Patient

"I have shared the podium with my good friend Dr. Ed. The two of us—a cancer doc and a veterinarian, an unlikely tag team—understand the amazing healing power of the animal-human connection and have devoted our careers to this bond. I am delighted that, finally, medical doctors embrace the importance of our companion animals as a key part of the pet prescription. Dr. Ed explains this connection and devotes nearly a full chapter to the power of the 'Lab' results and 'cat' scan in modern medicine in his outstanding book about prevention and survival."

Marty Becker, D.V.M., Veterinary Correspondent
for the American Humane Association,
founding member of Core Team Oz for *The Dr. Oz Show*,
best-selling author and advocate for the healing power of pets

"Forget the TV doctors (please!). Dr. Ed Creagan is the real deal, a superb physician who knows what it takes for people to live long and well. In this book, he generously shares his experience and wisdom with the rest of us. I, for one, am taking his guidance to heart, and I hope to outlive him!"

Ira Byock, M.D., Professor, Geisel School of Medicine
at Dartmouth, palliative care physician, and
author of *Dying Well* and *The Best Care Possible*

"I saw Dr. Creagan at Mayo Clinic for a life-threatening condition thirty years ago. We looked at my prognosis and prayed, and then we got busy surviving. Sometimes the best medicine—besides a battalion of medical care—is a doctor who is kind, gracious, and understanding. That's Dr. Creagan. I thank God for His help, but I also thank Dr. Creagan for helping me survive a scary diagnosis. He says I'm a miracle. And I am."

Candy Wood Lindley,
author of *Face of Faith: Discovering a Different Kind of Makeover*

"Dr. Creagan's gracious advice and support were instrumental in developing A Time to Heal, our holistic rehabilitation program for cancer survivors. As a physician, Ed is top notch, but more importantly, he recognizes the human issues involved in health problems. His compassion and genuine care for people make it possible for him to address the whole person and not just the disease."

Stephanie Koraleski, Ph.D., CEO, *A Time to Heal*

How ^{NOT} to Be My Patient

A Physician's Secrets for Staying Healthy
and Surviving Any Diagnosis

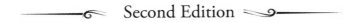 Second Edition

Edward T. Creagan, M.D., F.A.A.H.P.M.

Mayo Clinic Medical Oncologist/Cancer Specialist
and Palliative Care Consultant
John and Roma Rouse Professor of Humanism in Medicine
Professor of Medical Oncology

with Sandra Wendel

WRITE ON INK
PUBLISHING

How Not to Be My Patient and the information contained in this book are not intended as a substitute for the advice and/or medical care of the reader's physician, nor are they meant to discourage or dissuade the reader from seeking the advice of his or her physician. The reader should regularly consult with a physician on matters relating to his or her health, and especially with regard to symptoms that may require diagnosis. Any eating or lifestyle regimen should be undertaken under the direct supervision of the reader's physician. If the reader has any questions concerning the information presented in this book, or its application to his or her particular medical profile, or if the reader has unusual medical or nutritional needs or constraints that may conflict with the advice of this book, he or she should consult his or her physician. If the reader is pregnant or nursing, she should consult her physician before embarking on any nutrition or lifestyle program.

Neither the authors nor the publisher shall be liable or responsible for any loss or damage allegedly arising as a consequence of the reader's use or application of any information or suggestions in this book.

The cases described in this book are not those of actual patients, but rather reflect a composite of situations that Dr. Edward T. Creagan has dealt with in the course of his professional life.

This book reflects the individual views and opinions of Dr. Edward T. Creagan and does not necessarily reflect those of the Mayo Clinic.

Library of Congress Cataloging-in-Publication Data
Creagan, Edward T.
    How not to be my patient: a physician's secrets for staying healthy and surviving any diagnosis / Edward T. Creagan with Sandra Wendel.
        p. cm.
    Includes bibliographical references and index.
    1. Health 2. Cancer—Prevention. 3. Diagnosis. I. Wendel, Sandra.
    II. Title.
    Paperback ISBN: 978-0-9916544-1-3
    Mobi ISBN: 978-0-9916544-2-0
    EPUB ISBN: 978-0-9916544-3-7
    LCCN: 2014936155

Publisher: Write On Ink Publishing
                13518 L Street
                Omaha, NE 68137
                (402) 884-5995
                www.HowNotToBeMyPatient.com

10 9 8 7 6 5 4 3 2 1

*To my patients and their families
who have so heroically dealt with such a dreadful disease—cancer.*

Contents

Foreword

—❦—

Living Proof

AUTHOR'S NOTE:
First, a word from one of my patients.

Why am I wearing this yellow bracelet? It's not because I'm a Lance Armstrong fan; I wear it as a reminder of the deadly disease I once had and beat, just like Lance did. When people see the yellow band and ask me about it, their typical response to my answer is, "Wow, I never knew you had cancer." That's when I shock them even more by telling them I've beaten cancer twice.

In 1990, with just a couple of weeks left to my senior year of high school, I had a peculiar-looking mole removed from my left shoulder. The procedure was quick and simple. I thought nothing of it. Three days later, I was meeting with an oncologist to go over the pathology report.

The cancer specialist told me I had malignant melanoma, one of the deadliest forms of skin cancer. The doctor seemed optimistic because we'd caught the cancer early. Surgery was scheduled for the week after graduation.

The procedure was relatively quick, only taking an hour or so. All I really remember about it was waking up before the procedure was done and asking the nurse if we could order a pizza. Needless to say, the doctor was not amused or happy with his anesthesiologist.

With the surgery behind me, and the oncologist confirming that reoccurrence would be rare, my outlook was good.

Round 2 came a little over a year later. I had developed a pain under my left arm. The cancer had spread to my lymph nodes.

Without any hesitation my oncologist pushed the red button and said, "This kid's going to Mayo."

After the surgery to remove the baseball-sized tumor in my armpit, it was now time to review the results with my new oncologist at Mayo Clinic. Dr. Edward Creagan walked into my hospital room and introduced himself, then wanted to know what I liked to do, where I was going to school, and so on. He was more interested in my life than any doctor I'd ever met.

Instead of talking about the results from the surgery and what lay ahead for me, we talked about me and what made me tick. He had such a sense of calm and reassurance that I almost forgot I was sick. He showed not only compassion but concern for me in the true sense of a caregiver.

And then we talked about the news: He said I had a 95 percent chance of the cancer showing up again in less than a year, but exactly where and when, no one knew. Not exactly reassuring news and less-than-desirable odds.

After leaving the clinic the first time, I had a million thoughts and fears going through my head. *Is this the beginning of the end?* My first odds were highly in my favor, and I lost. This time the odds were stacked against me, giving me almost no chance of beating them. *Would I be back in a month? A year? Where would the cancer spread next? Would I be able to live a productive life, or would this disease hinder me from enjoying the things in life that I loved so much (water sports, hockey, hunting, athletics)?*

After a day or two of really worrying about what could happen, I decided that was no way to go through life. I told myself that I would live my life as if I'd never had cancer and never would; despite the staggering odds, I told myself I would beat them. I wasn't going to let this ugly disease beat me.

Fast forward 23 years, countless tests, scans, X-rays, and every other test known to medicine—and more than 40 trips to Mayo Clinic—I continue to be free of cancer.

Although I now live quite some distance from Rochester, Minnesota, I still make the trip every year to get my checkup and clean bill of health from Dr. Creagan. I could visit my local medical center, but it's worth the whole trip when Dr. Creagan walks through the door with a smile on his face and immediately reassures me that everything is okay, all tests are good.

Each time I see Dr. Creagan I'm reminded of how special life is, and I thank my lucky stars that I'm here. He always lifts me up and helps me see the important things in life: my kids, family, friends, and conscious, healthy lifestyle.

My visits with Dr. Creagan always seem to open my eyes a little wider and make me feel better about myself and thankful for all that I have going for me. I won't lie to you and tell you that I never worry about going in for a checkup and having him tell me they've found something, but very rarely do I dwell on the cancer that I had back in the early 1990s. It may seem somewhat odd, but I am lucky to be his patient.

—Chris Peterson

Introduction

We are each put on this planet
to do something that no one else can do quite as well as we can.

"He has cancer," they would whisper with pity and dread. The residents of my grandmother's rooming house would go to great lengths to avoid John G., the unemployed factory worker in room 212, as if somehow by just talking to him they would catch his horrible disease.

Most residents of 615 Hunterdon Street were down-and-outers, renting rooms by the day, week, or month. Most were unemployed, but a few worked at a neighboring bar called the PON, Pride of Newark (a sure contradiction in terms), if they weren't on the other side of the bar battling with the bottle.

Having cancer in 1952 was as close to a death sentence as awaiting the electric chair from prison's death row—perhaps faster. What we didn't know then about cancer could fill volumes. But for me, a precocious second-grader living with my Irish immigrant grandmother who owned the 22-room boarding house in the Ironbound section of Newark, New Jersey, being around someone with cancer was a defining moment—maybe not in medical history but in mine.

You see, the gentleman in room 212 had a colostomy, in which his bowels emptied into a bag on the outside of his body because colon cancer had destroyed part of his intestine. I was able to comfortably change his appliance (bag) and simply knew that I would care for people like this for the rest of my life. That was the way it was. No debate. No discussion. I just knew. This was my first experience with cancer. I was eight years old.

My first clinical encounter was as a second-year medical student at New York Medical College. The year was 1968. I was assigned an elderly woman with advanced cancer of the stomach. Sunken eyes, hollow cheeks, skin stretched over bare bones; she was a living cadaver. When I first walked onto the ward and saw her, I thought she was dead. But I found the courage to approach her bedside.

Who was this woman? Did she have a family? What made her laugh or cry? What biological nightmare brought her to this dismal fate? I found it intriguing—fascinating in a morbid way—that one cell went haywire, robbed her of her future, and eventually resulted in her death. She had no chance for a reprieve.

How did this happen? I was "hooked" on the journey to find answers to the cancer question. My classmates thought I was crazy to deliberately seek out the cancer patients. It was hopeless, they said. I was wasting my time and efforts. They were wrong.

A Disease of the Soul

I was initially attracted to the biology and the genetics of cancer and was intrigued with the notion of mixing various types of chemotherapy (chemicals used for treatment), then adding radiation and immune-related treatments. But it was soon obvious to me that my attraction was not a fascination with cancer as a disease of the body but cancer as a disease of the soul.

Over these past four decades, I have pursued a path chosen years earlier in a grungy rooming house helping a sick and sad old man. Through him and the 40,000 other encounters with cancer patients I've worked with at one of the world's foremost medical centers, I have discovered the majesty and the resiliency of the human spirit. I learn from my patients. I listen to their stories. And I learn to treat each day as a gift. A day not to be wasted.

In effect, the oncologist (the cancer specialist) becomes the spiritual leader—priest, minister, rabbi, for example—for patients and their families. I'd estimate that at least 70 percent of our time is spent simply listening to patients and hearing their stories, rather than dripping toxic chemicals into their bodies.

As a physician, I'm inspired to hear the survival skills and tactics of patients who are at risk of being crushed by life's unfairness. It is their 11th hour. And no governor is standing by on the hotline to commute their sentences. Those stories keep me going.

Every cancer patient is surrounded by a litany of emotional nightmares: the prodigal son who does not return; the wayward daughter who reluctantly returns home; the mortgage that is never paid off; the business reversals, shattered dreams, and missed opportunities (especially the chance to say, "I'm sorry" or "Forgive me").

The most painful words I hear far too often at the bedside are these: "I will never know how good I could have been. Maybe I could have made the big time, and now there is no time left." Yet, somehow, these patients continue to thrive and are a tremendous source of courage and admiration.

What I have learned from them is not to sweat the small stuff, but rather to savor each moment, to grasp it firmly, and to try to make the world a little better than it is right now. For me, each patient is a gift to be cherished.

We physicians need to understand that each patient is a person with a past and a present, a life spent dealing with a dreaded diagnosis.

Out of Suffering Comes Wisdom

The oncologist has "defining moments" every day if he or she takes the time to listen. Everybody has a drama. If we have patience, we doctors can come to know the human spirit.

We are each put on this planet to do something that no one else can do quite as well as we can. The lesson from thousands of patients is that everyone has a story. The overarching need of every human being is for recognition and acknowledgment. We want to be listened to, not preached at. We each say, in a special way, *Make me feel important. I am unique.*

Someone once said that everyone has at least one story good enough for a book, and perhaps this is mine. I wrote this book so that you can avoid cancer and other dreaded diseases. You have control over your destiny. You can and must take charge. As a patient, your job is to become the most empowered, the most knowledgeable person about your disease, because you are in charge of your decisions about treatment. No one has a greater stake in your health than you do. The buck stops with you, not your doctor.

"You're the doctor," some patients say to me, implying that I should advise them what to do. "No," I tell them. "You are the patient, you are in charge. Together, we will take this journey."

Sometimes, together, as doctor and patient, we may have to look at the relative futility of trying to treat advanced disease with current treatment plans. Many cancer treatments may worsen quality of life, and patients need to understand this reality. But let me be perfectly clear: For some cancers, and other diseases, the track record with current treatment is positive and hopeful and holds the potential for cure.

Let me share an amazing story. It was 1983. I had the privilege of evaluating a 56-year-old man for advanced lung cancer. He was referred to me from a prestigious medical institution in the Midwest. When I asked him what he was told about his illness there, he said, "They told me to pick out a good blue suit and six pallbearers."

He has returned to see me once a year every year since then. He has the same blue suit. Five of the six pallbearers are dead, and his original oncologist is in a nursing home. He always asks me how I am doing. Astonishing! He has lived with cancer, and he asks me how I'm doing!

This is what keeps us cancer specialists coming back.

How Not to Be My Patient

I inherited my father's fascination with the Sport of Kings— thoroughbred racing—and eagerly await the arrival of the Triple Crown. Most of us know the names of some of these three races: the Kentucky Derby, the greatest two minutes in sports; the Preakness; and the Belmont Stakes, the 1.5-mile route in New York that often signals the end of many thoroughbreds' careers.

I learned a lot at the track—far more than from any courses in sociology. The betting game comes with its own set of rules. The weekend gambler might just as well throw his money into the wind without some knowledge of the horses, the riders, the trainers, and the tracks. There is no such thing as luck. At the track we may lose money. The medical game is played the same way but with higher stakes. In medicine, we may lose our life or our quality of life.

Consumers of health care need to understand how the game is played. Medicine is at the crossroads. There are presently 79 million baby boomers marching in lockstep cadence into their 60s and 70s, who will place crushing pressures on the health care system during their older years. National changes with the Affordable Care Act on the health insurance side of the equation are evolving as we speak.

I am hardly a health care economist, but in the current climate the fees doctors get from Medicare do not fully cover the cost of providing the service. Mayo Clinic reports megamillion-dollar losses. Imagine the losses your medical clinic is taking. These deficits are not fiscally sustainable, so some health care organizations have limited their access for patients covered by Medicare. Some clinics have informed these patients that effective as of a certain date, they may be forced to pay cash for services.

Add those challenges to the issues patients face trying to get medical care. Sure, if you have crushing chest pain and go to the emergency room in a major metropolitan area, most likely you will get excellent care. But if you have a routine, nagging concern, you may have great frustration just getting an appointment.

You may not see a doctor but a "mid-level provider," such as a nurse-practitioner or physician assistant. Each plays an important role in medicine. However, the sands of time are shifting, and medical care, as we know it, is quickly fading from the scene.

We as patients need to understand the changing nature of medical students. Most are women, and it's highly unlikely that most of them will practice full-time. But now for the really serious news. About 95 percent of medical students are not going into primary care or general internal medicine or family medicine; they are specializing. So the boots are simply not on the ground to care for us when we have a problem.

Another part of this drama is much less publicized. Bureaucratic strangleholds on medicine and a bewildering number of regulations are driving physicians to retire at younger ages and at higher rates than ever before. If you doubt me, ask your doctor, especially if he or she is older than 50. Large numbers of patients need care. Fewer physicians are available to deliver care. And patients are bombarded with information on the Internet. What's a person to do?

Your Best Bet—The Daily Double

Here's the inside track. An ounce of prevention is still well worth a pound of treatment. As we head into an environment of cost containment and the ratcheting down of access to medical services, you need every scrap of sound medical information you can get to truly be in charge of your own health and longevity. Your best daily double against cancer and other serious diseases is still healthy lifestyle choices and early detection of disease. But there's much more.

Let's look at the odds: more patients flooding the exam rooms, a greater number of older patients putting pressure on a health care system with a dwindling number of doctors, regulations and low reimbursements from insurance programs forcing doctors to retire, and changes in the insurance and government program payments.

We as patients need to be savvy consumers because we will be buying our own coverage, and we need to understand what we need as patients and what we do not need. Marcus Welby, M.D., is no longer in practice, and we need to know how the game is played—or we lose. The best approach: stay fit, medically wise, and know your options because the "system" is still shaking out, and you can get lost and overwhelmed with life-and-death decisions.

Ideally, each patient and family has a primary care provider to be the medical quarterback. But less than 5 percent of medical school graduates enter primary care. All the other doctors in training are specializing. Why? I have connected with wonderful physicians in training over the last several decades. They are dedicated and compassionate; but they are concerned about lifestyle issues, and so they are less willing to have medicine become the primary life focus that it was for my generation who graduated medical school in the 1970s.

I vividly recall spending my days off in the emergency room of an inner-city hospital in New York in order to gain extra clinical experience. Few learners would do that today, and perhaps that is healthier.

Another issue: the primary care provider has more stress and burnout and less income than the specialists, so fewer learners enter this area of medicine. It's an economic, time-and-money decision.

I'm going to share with you how to make the best choices, the most important medical decisions, you will ever make in your life. And I'm not talking about track tips or stock tips. By the time I see most of my patients, they have weeks, not months, left to live. Let there be no doubt: They are courageous, and we have many, many success stories that defy what we know about cancer. But truth be known, about half of my patients never needed to walk into my exam room because their cancers were related to lifestyle choices they made along the way.

I'm not placing blame or guilt. There is little merit in looking back. I'm telling you the reality. The number 1 fear of the person on the street is not heart disease, AIDS, or arthritis. It is cancer. Public speaking is a close second, I am told. I can't tell you how to stand up in front of a crowd. But in this book, I will tell you what you can do, for yourself and your family, so you won't ever be my patient.

Although we cannot prevent all cancers and all scary diseases, we can place ourselves "on the rail," in a position to make the final sprint to the finish line. A guarantee? Of course not, but what I learned at my father's side at the track is that we can shift the odds in our favor if we have the knowledge to be proactive and involved in the most important race of our lives.

You can bet on it.

In these pages, I will relate many stories about some of the most incredible people I have ever met. I want you to meet them too. But because of my deepest respect for their privacy and because of my legal obligation as a doctor to preserve the doctor-patient confidentiality bond, you will not be given, nor do you need, all the details about each of these remarkable patients. They are real. Their stories are real. And without them, I could not make this journey with you.

PART ONE

What Your Doctor
Never Tells You

1

The Race Against Time

We never know what the future will bring,
but we do know that the future belongs
to the fit and to the focused.
The best way to predict the future is to create the future.

My father had a serious medical condition. He had an aversion to something called gainful employment. Intrigued with numbers and horses, he was convinced that there were reasonably predictable patterns governing why some horses won races and some did not.

He parlayed this passion into a career as a professional handicapper. He spoke in the argot of the shadowy world of the track. Terms such as *speed ratings, track variants, post-position bias, blinkers, run-down bandages, maiden claimers, routers, sprinters,* and *bug boys* were factored into decisions of whether to bet or not to bet.

As a young boy, I spent many days at his side in pari-mutuel palaces with such exotic names as Pimlico, Hialeah, Saratoga, Tropical, and Gulfstream Park. I learned a lot of life's great lessons at the track. But one lesson that stuck with me in my later years as a physician has been the most valuable: Don't bet blindly.

Casual bettors at the track will consistently lose shirts, drawers, and big bucks, all because they lack some understanding of the *Daily Racing Form*. This arcane publication contains reams of data on past performances of horses. My father did understand this. It's why he was a success. I never remember him working elsewhere, but I do remember him driving new Cadillacs and wearing $600 suits with $100 ties (and never graduating from high school).

This may sound far removed from the exam room at Mayo Clinic where I see patients from all over the world, but it isn't.

Every day that you live, you risk your future by what you do. Or, in the case of most people, you risk your future by what you *don't* do. If you understand the odds, you can shift them in your favor. You cannot be a casual gambler. You must understand how the game is played.

None of us is guaranteed a future. You could drop dead tomorrow. Or you may live to 105—even if you smoke, drink, eat anything you want, and rarely move from your Barcalounger. But, as my father would say, that's a long shot. Yes, long shots do pay off, but not as often as smart bets do.

How can you go where the smart money goes when it comes to your health? That's what this chapter is all about.

It's amazing to me that so many people bet on their futures unwisely by ignoring the health risks they engage in. Or they know the risks and hope for an unlikely payoff. Are you betting you'll be that one of a hundred or a thousand who lives long and healthfully— perhaps even reaching the age of 100—despite your avoiding the behaviors that are known to enhance health?

Many of the people I see in the exam room lose this bet. Yes, genetics and inheritance need to be considered, but lifestyle choices play a decisive role in whether you will develop major diseases. If a jockey or trainer gave you the inside scoop on a race, you'd plunk down your money without thinking. Let me help you make a wise bet on your health. Even my dad would say the surest bet remains an ounce of prevention.

Know your health risks and make smart choices. I'll help you stay on the rail and close fast at the finish. It's your future you're gambling on. The smart money is on the right choices.

My Prescription for Survival

As Americans, we focus on high-tech toys to solve medical problems. The CT scan, the MRI, and the PET scan help detect disease at its earliest and most treatable stage, and in doing so, these tests help people hold off the aging process. Could life everlasting be just down the road?

Technology is not enough. What's the proof? People in countries with some of the lowest availability of scans and other high-tech gadgets have better health care and longer life spans than we do.

The spectacular popularity of medications, such as Viagra to treat male impotence and Propecia to put hair back on our heads, is evidence that we are increasingly focused on lifestyle medications designed to make us healthy and happy. Botox injections are wiping the ravages of age from our faces. If we just pump enough antioxidants into ourselves, we can surely fend off the free radicals racing around inside our bodies and making us old. Or can we?

Is this the secret to living longer and aging better? Where did this attitude come from?

Although the point is debatable, the eradication of polio through the Salk vaccine gave Americans the notion that big government, big industry, and big universities would provide the panacea to put the genie of illness back in the bottle. Unfortunately, we as a society have missed the boat. We have bet on the wrong horse.

We're demanding drugs for conditions that aren't even illnesses. Is pregnancy and childbirth a disease? How about jet lag, menopause, or erectile dysfunction? Aging and baldness? Are our anxieties about these "nondiseases" siphoning resources away from real medical issues?

We need to embrace the cold realities of life, work life, and modern medicine so that we can devise a survival kit for ourselves and our families. Since when is aging or baldness considered an illness? We have plenty of diagnostic codes without adding road rage or loneliness. These could be symptoms of a society sick and tired of being sick and tired. These could be symptoms of a society fixated on smaller problems while missing the boat on big health issues.

Here's my prescription for survival: We each need to take personal responsibility for our own health and welfare in order to decrease our risks of developing disease, especially cancer. Let me explain. Most experts now acknowledge that at least half of all people die early because of illness caused by lifestyle choices, dietary factors, and behavioral patterns. In other words, what you do and don't do with your body will kill you faster. You can lower your risk for premature death and disability right now—it's never too late.

And for those whose future includes an encounter with a life-threatening illness, such as cancer or heart disease or diabetes, there is no doubt in my mind: People who are physically fit, spiritually focused, psychologically intact, and who have a support system do far better with their illnesses than those who are isolated and disenfranchised.

The Best Medicine Is No Medicine at All

Mounting evidence from sociologists, psychologists, and medical researchers suggests that strong social support—I like the term *connectedness* —can help you live longer. I know this to be true because I see the wonders of family and friends and pets every day with my patients.

A study of Harvard graduates from the classes of 1941 and 1944 identified the following common keys to a long, healthy life. These were men (yes, mostly men at Harvard then) who became some of the most prominent policy makers, educators, scientists, and corporate leaders in our country. Those who remained productive through their 70s and 80s shared these characteristics:

- They had stable, long-term relationships and marriages.
- Through weight management and exercise, they maintained an ideal body weight.
- They had moderate alcohol use, if they chose to drink.
- Regular exercise was part of their lives—and this was at a time before the benefits of exercise were really promoted.
- They developed adaptive coping skills, such as a sense of humor and resilience, and were able to refocus their energies on art, music, and other activities.

Social involvement and resiliency are the most powerful predictors of living healthy as you age. We can also learn from the people living on the isolated island of Okinawa. The Okinawans live an average of 15 years longer than we Americans do. Considering their lack of medical technology, they practically live forever.

For one thing, they are not obsessed with nondiseases. They eat a low-calorie diet. They engage in regular physical activity, drink moderate amounts of alcohol, and, most important, they develop strong social networks and spiritual beliefs that foster a sense of well-being. Sounds too simple to be true.

This is not rocket science. This is human nature.

I hope you're seeing the pattern here. Work at something you enjoy, and you'll probably live long enough to cash in your 401(k), buy the lake home, see your grandchildren grow up, travel the seven seas, or cross the country in an RV. Attitude matters. Pessimists die, on average, eight years younger than people who have a positive outlook on life. And if patients with lung cancer have a good quality of life, they live longer than patients with a poorer quality of life.

We were designed to be joyful and fun-filled individuals. Do you enjoy eating dinner with a grouch or playing golf under the doom and gloom of a Chicken Little personality? If you cannot have fun or generate joy for yourself and others around you, you will have little incentive to go the distance in the race of life.

Every one of us has things we like to do and are good at doing. Cultivate and nurture these interests to make life fulfilling and promising.

You can't just wake up one day, however, and see the world in a better light (or put this book down and miraculously have a new attitude just because I suggested it). But engaging in positive social activities will transform you. I guarantee it.

My 8 Commandments for Living Long and Living Well

1. Form stable long-term relationships. Friends, families, colleagues, even pets, are clearly buffers against stress. Rarely does the isolated, marginalized person go the distance.
2. Maintain ideal body weight. Many of us struggle with obesity, and the health fallout is significant in terms of high blood pressure, diabetes, arthritis, and stroke. Ideal body weight doesn't mean starving yourself to look like something out of a fashion magazine, but it means eating sensibly considering your height, heredity, and lifestyle.

3. Eat a plant-based diet with an emphasis on green leafy vegetables, six to eight servings of fruit each day, fish and poultry rather than red meat (in moderation), and pay attention to unsaturated fats, such as olive and canola oil. You don't have to be a brown rice-and-tofu vegetarian. Again, being sensible makes sense here.
4. Engage in regular physical activity. Let the experts debate about whether 30 minutes is best or 60 minutes is better. Just get active doing what you do every day, and throw in a walk four or five times a week.
5. Longevity does not allow for smoking. Enough said.
6. Use alcohol in moderation, if at all. Although there is some evidence that a glass of red wine (4 oz.) may be protective against certain types of heart disease, alcohol consumption can be harmful to many other conditions.
7. Foster a sense of spirituality, a sense of connectedness to nature or your higher power or some force or factor over and above yourself.
8. Find meaning and purpose in life. This is your reason to push on even in the face of adversity. What gets you up in the morning? A paycheck is not enough.

It's a balancing act: You won't live forever, but you can't live like there's no tomorrow, because tomorrow is coming. You can prepare for tomorrow today by making smart lifestyle choices or changing poor health habits—it's never too late to do that.

When you make the right choices, you can take a licking and keep on ticking, even when life throws you a curve ball, literally. Let me tell you a story: My wife, Peggy, plays women's softball. She's years older than her teammates, but because she's a vigorous woman who is careful about what she eats and runs religiously, she's fit and healthy.

One hot summer night, a pop fly was hit to her in left field. She dogged the ball and was on it, but lost it in the lights. Instead of ducking for cover, she thought she had her glove at least close—

until the elusive ball whacked her in the nose. She fell to the ground, seriously injured.

Seven hours later, after extensive emergency reconstructive surgery, she was bruised and hurting, looking like a raccoon with her two black eyes, but alive and healing quickly. I attribute her recovery in part to skilled emergency crews, and to equally skilled surgeons, but, most of all, to her healthy mind and body being able to take a punch and bounce back.

The same would be true for any life-threatening illness. The fitter you are, the better you will be able to withstand the curve ball that comes your way. And, frankly, my own level of fitness stood me in great stead the night Peggy was injured because I was 250 miles away, preparing to speak the next day at a wellness conference, when the call came from the ER at 3:00 a.m. telling me Peggy was going into surgery.

Jarred from sleep by the call nobody wants to get in the middle of any night, I was packed and out of the hotel in minutes, headed back to Rochester on dark two-lane roads for the longest drive of my life. But because I was healthy and in shape, I had the emotional and physical stamina needed to make sound decisions—and a long drive in the wee hours of the night—in the midst of crisis.

We never know what the future will bring, but we do know that the future belongs to the fit and to the focused.

Live Long Enough to Cash In Your 401(k)

The big day has finally arrived. Your boss shakes your hand and wishes you well. Your colleagues gather around a cake and make small talk about landing the big fish in your retirement, or joke about what you'll do now that you don't have to come to the office.

A cardboard box is filled with the contents of your desk: your family pictures, desktop trinkets, snowball paperweight, and stale candy. Your twentysomething replacement has all but moved in on your accounts. Your name is off the cubicle, and you wonder what you'll do for the next 30 years.

One more stop: the benefits office.

In a few minutes, you will be asked to make one of the most significant and far-reaching financial decisions of your life: How do you want to receive your pension?

What does this have to do with your health?

Plenty. Because before you can make any decision about your pension distribution, you need to seek the guidance of skilled individuals, such as an accountant, a certified financial planner, a tax adviser, an attorney, and—believe it or not—a doctor.

Let's suppose you are generally healthy, with normal blood pressure, no diabetes or heart disease, and your mother lived to a ripe old age. For you, the annuity of a fixed amount every month becomes a reasonable option. You could very well "outlive" the lump sum option you are presented along with the gold watch—and laugh all the way to the bank.

On the other hand, you may have a serious medical condition, such as cancer, and let's suppose that your expected survival is limited to a year or two.

In that situation, a reasonable option would be door number 2, the lump sum. You and your family would work with professionals to set investments in motion to take care of your family, despite the ups and downs of Wall Street.

Retirement decisions are not always as obvious as this example. And who gets a pension these days? Very few of us. But you will be making decisions about when to take Social Security and when to tap into your 401(k).

From a practical standpoint, however, I suggest you see your doctor around the time your retirement is planned. Some minor blood abnormalities or trivial symptoms might lead to a CT scan or EKG, and then to a diagnosis of a life-threatening illness. In that case, your financial options would be clear. You may not be around long enough to collect your full pension, but you can make provisions for your family.

Life is complicated and not always fair. But before you sign on the dotted line, understand your health—and the rules of trusts and sound financial planning.

Oh, Boy, Health Care Delivery Is Changing

Once upon a time, when life was simple and we were not whipsawed by the digital age, we went to see, typically, a primary care physician—the Marcus Welby of the neighborhood—who knew us and our family and cared for us. And sometimes the doctor made house calls. He (most doctors then were male) had relatively limited medical treatments in that black bag, and technology was unheard of. But the doctor not only listened with a stethoscope, the doctor listened to us, talked about our families, and provided some simple recommendations. Usually, we got better.

Insurance normally covered the cost of services, or there was a cash payment (or barter). But with technology in the exam room in the form of CT scans and MRIs and electronic medical records, everything changed. And if you don't have insurance, you are at a profound disadvantage.

We are now in the midst of the "perfect storm" for delivery of health care. *The Perfect Storm* was a book by Sebastian Junger outlining a disastrous storm off the coast of New England that sank a fishing vessel with its crew. Maybe you saw the movie starring George Clooney and Mark Wahlberg.

The once-in-a-century storm was a combination of wind speed, temperature, and water temperature that created monstrous waves and freezing temperatures.

As patients and consumers of health care, we are now in the eye of the perfect storm of medicine. Let me explain the three key factors coming together in this perfect storm.

First, patients are becoming older and sicker. Simply walk through any hospital or emergency room, and you can clearly see the aging of the American population. Not surprisingly, the elderly patient requires more complicated and more sophisticated medical care. With the boomers joining their aging parents, we will see an unprecedented number of older patients needing care.

And what do more patients need? More doctors. My second point is this: There has been a dramatic shift in the health care provider community. Once upon a time, graduates of medical schools usually went into general specialties, such as internal medicine or surgery. However, almost all graduates now head into highly technical subspecialties, such as ophthalmology or orthopedic surgery.

There are data from American medical schools that more than 95 percent of graduates will enter some narrow focus of expertise, rather than general internal medicine or general surgery or family practice. This means that we as patients will have a limited number of physicians upon whom we can call if we should have a serious medical problem.

And I'm sad to say that my medical colleagues are experiencing burnout and stress in unprecedented numbers. Many attribute their burnout to the changing health care delivery system, pressure from insurers to see more patients in the day, lower rates of reimbursement from Medicare and Medicaid, and the fear of malpractice suits. So wonderful clinicians are bailing out of medicine altogether, and I discuss how to spot a doc who may be under excess stress and strain and how to deal with that in this book.

Suffice to say here, burnout removes doctors from the delivery side of medicine at a time when we need more, not fewer, general practitioners—and probably a good number of geriatric specialists for our seniors.

The third issue in this perfect storm is hardly news. Consider the devastating costs of health care. Every reader of this book has some nightmare story of a friend or family member or coworker pushed to the brink of bankruptcy because of escalating health care costs.

Here's an example. A medicine called Yervoy (or ipilimumab) is one of the first FDA-approved medications for the treatment of malignant melanoma (black-mole cancer). The medication consists of an intravenous infusion once every three weeks for three or four treatments. Although the price may vary by part of the country, in general, the bill is approximately $120,000, and that often does not include the costs of treating the patient's complications, which could require a hospital stay.

Regardless of how airtight insurance policies are, no policy covers every expense, and even a small percentage of this bill can be devastating. Obviously, there is a tremendous economic incentive to stay well, but an equally important incentive is quality of life and sense of well-being. No one can afford to get sick.

We each need to understand that we are competing for a seat at the health care table. And with the aging of the American population, that seat is going to become dreadfully crowded.

According to the New England Centenarian study, the most rapidly increasing population segment in America today is that of individuals over age 100. In the early 20th century, the typical American had a survival of about 45 years. In some communities today, that survival figure is 80 to 90. And, if we are in an affluent area with access to health care, it is not surprising that many individuals may well live to be 100. Just think for a moment what the pressures on the health care system will be with that scenario.

Futurists are predicting radical changes coming, such as medical treatments that can slow or stop the aging process, according to a Pew Research Center study in 2013. Can the life span be extended to 120? Maybe. Yet adults in this survey said an ideal life span would be between 79 and 100 years.

Is 90 the new 85?

In 1980, there were 720,000 people aged 90 and older in the United States. In 2010, there were 1.9 million people aged 90 and older. By 2050, the ranks of people 90 and older may reach 9 million, according to a report from the U.S. Census Bureau, commissioned by the National Institute on Aging.

Why are these people defying the odds? A study from the Albert Einstein College of Medicine interviewed hundreds of centenarians. Longevity genes, they said in the *Journal of the American Geriatrics Society*, may be more important than lifestyle and behavior when it comes to living an exceptionally long life.

An average person who has lived to 90 years of age has a life expectancy today of 4.6 more years (versus 3.2 years in 1929), while those who pass the century mark are projected to live another 2.3 years.

The majority of those 90 years and older reported having one or more limitations in physical function. Two-thirds had difficulty with such activities as walking or climbing stairs.

Women 90 years and older outnumber men nearly 3 to 1.

What does this mean for you? Will Grandma find a place to live with you? Is caregiving for aging parents in your future? Will you even want to retire early if you're healthy and intending to live another third of your life? Have you saved for retirement and beyond? What can you do now to keep from having disabilities when you are older?

The Demise of Doctors

Since Marcus Welby and the local family physician are rapidly disappearing, each of us needs to understand that we need an access point into the system. The emergency room or the urgent care center is a very inefficient and unsatisfactory way to deliver health care. Usually, there is little relationship with the health care provider in those situations. The facilities are not equipped for long-term care or any personal relationship. What should you do?

As we head deeper into the 21st century, much of health care will be provided by the "mid-level providers." Most of us find that term rather offensive, as these are credentialed colleagues who are the boots on the ground in delivering health care. They're often referred to by the terms physician assistant (P.A.) or nurse-practitioner (N.P.).

Most of these colleagues, depending on state regulations, have a bachelor's degree and then have the equivalent of a master's degree consisting of approximately 800 to 900 hours of clinical supervision.

They are wonderful colleagues who provide excellent care under difficult circumstances. In some medical centers, these colleagues have a narrow focus of specialization; for example, a P.A. might deal only with patients with cardiac disease or with breast cancer or infectious complications from surgery. An important take-home message is that we need to know who that person (P.A. or N.P. or something else) is, and how we can access that specialist in our moment of need.

You may find this mid-level provider in your current doctor's office. This is the team member who assists the overworked or unavailable physician.

Let's add another element to that perfect storm of an aging population, fewer doctors to treat them, and the rising cost of health insurance.

You can be assured that the next few years will see a "who's on first" scramble to figure out the health insurance coverage picture as preexisting conditions become covered, as health exchanges jockey to gain a foothold in the marketplace, as consumers and their employers weigh the coverage options and potential penalties, and as millions more Americans finally fall under the umbrella of "coverage."

Situations like the one I am about to tell you will become even more tricky. A beloved family member is a wonderful gentleman in his early 70s. He lives in a major metropolitan area and developed a complex neurological problem.

His primary care provider referred him to a surgeon who was "out of the network," meaning that the patient's insurance would not cover the cost of care by that surgeon. Yet he was uncomfortable with the recommendations of a doctor "in the network." So our patient was faced with a difficult decision. Does he undergo an expensive complicated surgery by a provider not within the system (this was his choice, and his outcome was excellent), or does he compromise his health by having care within the system but with a doctor who is perhaps less qualified. These are difficult decisions for patients and family members to understand.

So what is the final message from this early journey into the perfect storm brewing around health care? You must recognize the need to take responsibility for your own health, and I will expand on this countless times throughout the rest of this book.

You also need to be aware of the sweeping changes in the organization and the delivery of health care. Hardly a day goes by that there is not some comment in the media about mergers, acquisitions, and consolidations. Hospitals X, Y, and Z are swallowed up by some health care giant. What does that mean for you? You may lose that feeling of connectedness with your doctor, or your doc may be restricted in the tests he or she can order, and sometimes costs will increase.

Essential Keys to Long Life in a Changing World

We are now in the midst of one of the greatest migrations in the history of the world. Approximately 79 million post–World War II baby boomers are not only moving over the psychological aging hill they climbed 30 years ago, they're on the downhill side, looking hard at the diseases of aging. At the same time, their "Greatest Generation" parents are happily living longer—and not-so-happily experiencing the diseases of aging, as well.

With careful planning, these years can be creative and nurturing. But if left to chance and without planning, these years may not be productive at all. Let's look at our changing world and navigate our way to long life.

Key #1: You will live longer than your parents and their parents

If you are a woman age 50 and without active heart disease or cancer, you can expect to live into your 90s. However, the last 10 to 12 years of your life may well be spent living alone because men typically die at a much earlier age.

If you're a man and you make it to 65, you can expect at least 15 more years of life, and, with proper planning, these can be productive and creative times.

Midlife Americans at age 50 can expect to live another 30 years, according to an AARP report. That's almost nine years longer than your grandmother or great-grandmother lived if she was born in 1900. Although today's boomers may smoke less, which is contributing to longevity, they're more likely to be overweight. And obesity may take away any gains we've made in curbing smoking.

My message is this: Plan now, whatever your age, because you will probably live longer than your parents and their parents, and life is more fun when you're healthy enough to enjoy it. Disease is not inevitable. You're not "destined to die" of the same disease that prematurely took your mother. You're in control of your health destiny. And you can improve your health along the way.

Can you live forever? Probably not, even if you're cryogenically frozen, but researchers at Duke University say the maximum human life span will reach 100 in about six decades. Today's 65-year-old can expect to live another 17 years (for men) or 20 years (for women), according to Social Security life expectancy tables. Let's hope the Social Security Administration is holding your money for you!

What major diseases we worry about varies by age and background. But, in general, Americans fear cancer (41%), Alzheimer's (31%), heart disease (8%), stroke (8%), and diabetes (6%), according to a MetLife Foundation survey. Compare those fears to the leading causes of death (CDC):

- Birth to age 1: birth defects
- Age 1 to 44: unintentional injury/accidents
- Age 45 to 64: cancer
- Age 65 and up: heart disease

For the record, heart disease and stroke will kill more Americans than cancer and any of the other conditions combined. Half of all cancers can be attributed to lifestyle choices. Obesity plays into all these illnesses and raises the risk for all of them (cancer, heart disease, and diabetes). Obesity is becoming a serious health issue because rates have doubled in the past 20 years. Today, one-third of adults are overweight or obese, and one-sixth of children are. Unheard of and unprecedented. These children may not live as long as their parents because of these diseases.

This underscores the overarching importance of lifestyle issues and early detection to enhance our ability to diagnose and cure diseases of lifestyle.

My prescription for survival can help you live longer and better, but you must first address the issues that are holding you back. Prevention is, of course, my mantra, but I know that the behavior changes—even tiny ones—that lead to higher levels of health don't come easy.

In the next chapters, we'll examine whether you're ready to change, how to change, and what to focus on in the areas of exercise, nutrition, stress, habits (such as smoking and alcohol use), and sleep. We'll also look at other lifestyle choices you make every day, and find ways to get you moving toward wellness.

I'm not going to repeat the same tired messages you hear in the media. I take a little more unconventional approach to behavior change. For example, consider these questions that are answered in the chapters ahead:

- Do you know what the real Fountain of Youth is?
- What medicine is absolutely free?
- Do you know where to find the best nutritional choices in the grocery store?
- Is there room for fast food in your diet? (spoiler alert: yes)
- Why is some stress good for you?
- Do you know how to get the most out of your doctor visits?
- Why should you keep copies of your medical records?
- What is the best way to stay well in the hospital?
- What do long-term disease survivors know (that you need to know)?
- Can pets really keep you healthier?
- Why should you not believe the health headlines (most of the time)?

I'll fill you in on one of the secrets to living longer and healthier. It's health screening. Some medical tests are worth paying for; some are not. But, first, you must give your doctor a checkup. Like a good marriage, the doctor-patient relationship is critical to your health. Together, what you know about your body and your health will change your health behavior for the better. It's a partnership worth cultivating.

Key #2: You have to be a smart patient because doctors don't always know best—you do

When I was a young boy growing up in New Jersey, doctors not only seemed like old men, they *were* old men. Physicians would practice into their 70s. That would be almost unheard of now because of the threat of malpractice and the pace of technology. It is not at all uncommon to see physicians retiring in their 50s and heading off to the golf course or for careers far less stressful and more manageable, even concierge medicine where patients pay a fee for 24/7 access to the doc.

Today, the family doctor may not be there for us. Like his and her colleagues, the doc retired early and is on the first tee.

*Mis*managed care has taken choice out of our medical-care equation. In network, out of network, the search for Dr. Right usually takes us to a crowded waiting room with old magazines just to get our 16 minutes with a doctor who has three patients backed up and four calls holding on the phone—and a pager beeping.

Women are taking the lead in becoming empowered medical consumers. Women make 80 percent of the health care decisions (for themselves and their families) and are most likely to be the caregivers for their families, according to the Department of Labor. They also go to the doctor more often than men. Not surprisingly, 25 percent of my male counterparts had absolutely no doctor visits in 2011, according to the Centers for Disease Control and Prevention (CDC) figures (compared to 13 percent of women).

The Internet attempts to fill the information gap, but it often falls hopelessly short of providing trusted, actionable health answers. In fact, patients can fall into a worldwide web of snake oil if they're not sure how to navigate the murky waters of virtual medical hucksterism.

So where does this leave us? Welcome to the age of the empowered patient. You must learn to be your own best medical opinion because you are indeed calling the shots. In the next few chapters, I will tell you things your doctor never tells you. I will take you inside the medical world and tell you what doctors know and what they don't know. There is no magic or conspiracy "not to tell" patients what they need to know.

The system is tying our hands, cutting our time, piling up our paperwork, and leaving us little time for the real nitty-gritty of medicine—and that's eyeball time, "face time," with our patients. The laptop or tablet recording the electronic medical record often stands between the doctor and the patient.

You have to make us work for you. By being empowered, you can get the same medical information a doctor would give you under ideal circumstances; you just need to know what it all means—for your good health and the health of your family.

You'll find out how to get the best from your doctor visits. Why spend precious minutes talking about how much calcium you need, when you really want to discuss how tired you've been lately and whether those headaches mean anything? You'll learn why you need certain medical records with you at all times, which ones those are, and how to get them. Your medical records can be lifesaving if you know where they are and how you can get copies.

Like puzzle pieces that all fit together to form a big picture, your complete medical records can be invaluable when you're managing illness. Knowing where your records are and how to get them is your job these days. Don't leave it up to your doctor.

Where to turn for lifesaving health information is critical. Media hype and headlines can be misleading and downright wrong. In the chapters ahead, I discuss issues we were never taught in medical school. Medical breakthroughs and big-time cures are not taken lightly, and a study involving mice or even 14 people in Finland may eventually lead to medical enlightenment for you, but it's not likely soon.

So before you get your hopes up, put your guard up and learn to read between the lines when you hear about or read medical studies, especially on the Internet or cable news. I'll help you understand the medical headlines and teach you when to get excited and when to be skeptical.

Key #3: You can survive any diagnosis

The final section of this book tells you how to handle a serious diagnosis and even an acute emergency situation.

- You'll increase your odds of coming through if you know what to do first and how to take charge.
- If you can't take charge, you need to know how to call on a network of support for help.

I offer essential steps to making the best of any diagnosis—even if long-term survival is out of reach. But quality of life and a sense of peace and serenity are always within reach.

Whether they're trying to beat a difficult diagnosis or just searching for better medical care, patients frustrated with the medical "system" are increasingly seeking alternatives. Depending on the age group, up to half and more of us are currently using what would be termed complementary and alternative medical therapies: mind-body techniques, such as meditation; alternative medical systems, such as homeopathy and traditional Chinese medicine; biologically based substances, such as herbs and vitamins; body-based methods, including chiropractic; and energy therapies, such as therapeutic touch and Reiki.

As in any endeavor, the alternative medicine world can be its own worst enemy, fraught with the proverbial snake-oil salespeople and smoke and mirrors—only these days Dr. Scott's Magic Elixir is cleverly disguised as a vitamin or dietary "supplement" with enticing names, such as coral calcium, blue-green algae, and shark cartilage. You do have alternatives, and I will be among the first to discuss which work, which don't, and which might.

A Prescription That Works

We human beings are amazing creatures. With all forms of therapy, including the power of prayer, I've seen medical miracles among my patients. Things happen that go against everything I've ever learned in medical school.

Almost every day in the clinic, I see individuals who had dreadful prognoses based upon a pathology report, a CT scan, PET scan, or an operative report, yet they have continued to do amazingly well. A variety of sophisticated tests have been performed on these patients to find the key to their survival, and there does not seem to be a consistent theme from these studies. However, these patients do seem to have several traits in common.

I know this because I recently had the opportunity to review much of the world's literature on longevity and found three themes that seemed common to these long-term survivors:

A sense of religion. By this we mean individuals participating in the set of rules and regulations for certain belief systems, such as Catholicism, Judaism, Protestantism, or any of the world's religions. Others adhere to a less formal belief system or have their own sense of a higher power.

A sense of spirituality. There are many definitions for this term, but the one that seems to work for many individuals is the questioning of the ultimate purpose of life: Why are we here? What is this all about? It is an attempt to find meaning, purpose, and cohesion in a sea of chaos and confusion.

A sense of connectedness. These individuals typically have long-term meaningful adult relationships in terms of spouses or partners, or are members of a community that gives them support and encouragement during times of crisis.

Thirty-seven years ago, as a medical oncologist, I would see patients in their 70s, but that was most unusual. In the 1980s, I started to see patients in their 80s. Now it is not uncommon to see women—and men—in their 90s who are "dead fit," to use a racetrack term. They're candidates for aggressive surgery, radiation, and chemotherapy; whereas, years earlier, we never would have considered them strong enough.

When I meet with these amazing patients, I always inquire, "Tell me, Mrs. Smith or Mr. Jones, what is the secret of your youthful vitality?" First they laugh, embarrassed, and then answer, "I don't know." At this point, I jokingly offer to reduce their bill by 10 percent if they tell me. Then the stories unfold.

They all have a sense of meaning and purpose in life. They feel connected to someone or something, whether it's a person or a pet parakeet depending on them for their own purpose in life. They feel a need to contribute to society in some small way. Maybe they help a widow friend fill out her income tax forms or drive someone to the doctor or give advice to a granddaughter dealing with tough times. The final chapter gives you the inside track on survival and longevity, because successful aging does not happen by accident.

My Prevention Rx

Our population is aging at the same time that we're seeing fewer doctors in primary care and while costs continue to rise unabated. This perfect storm, along with massive changes in the health care delivery and health insurance system, will make seeing a doctor more difficult and more expensive. Enter the empowered patient: you. Nobody has a greater stake in your health than you do. Repeat after me …

Plan now, whatever your age, because you will probably live longer than your parents and their parents, and life is more fun when you're healthy enough to enjoy it, as I've said before. Disease is not inevitable. You're not "destined to die" of the same disease that prematurely took your mother, because you are more in control of your health destiny. But what can you do to improve your health along the way? A lot. That's why you're reading this book.

Do I have all the answers? Far from it. But let me tell you about a few people who have been helped by reading the earlier version of this book.

A few months ago, Peggy and I were visiting family in Colorado. In the airport I had a sense that a woman was looking at me. I was flattered, of course, but also surprised, as this rarely happens. She finally came over and asked if I were the doctor on the cover of the book.

I said I was. She explained how she had read this book, scheduled her mammogram, and stopped a small breast cancer early with surgery.

Another reader, a gentleman at the bank, came up to me as I waited in line to cash a check. He shared that his copy was dog-eared and on his nightstand. A stranger at dinner approached our table and asked for an autograph on a napkin, which I was delighted to provide. A few other readers have recognized me; we have shared stories and handshakes, even hugs. Patients often tell me they pray for me and my family.

I am truly honored by these gracious encounters, and I thank you for continuing to read.

2

Pack Your Own Parachute

Change doesn't come easy.
It's not always lasting.
But it's definitely worth a try.

The Biology of Living Longer and Better

Packing your own parachute is an important metaphor for survival. If you are jumping out of an airplane, whom would you trust with this life-preserving function? A loving companion? A trusted colleague? A close friend? Of course.

But the bottom line at the end of the day is clear: the buck stops with you. You need to pack your own parachute, and in this chapter I'll help you pack that parachute with lessons for health and wellness.

Just as we in the medical community suspected, your greatest health care expenses are driven by the lifestyle choices you make every day. My colleagues and I see the results of poor decision making every day in the clinic.

When researchers looked at the combined medical costs for thousands of employees of several major companies, they were surprised to see that the highest costs were for these conditions, from highest cost on down:

- Stress
- Depression
- Diabetes (blood sugar levels too high)

- Weight (too fat or too thin, but mostly being overweight or obese)
- Smoking (current or former smokers)
- Increased blood pressure
- Lack of exercise

These are easy targets. We can modify our behaviors and change our ways. But we don't. Why? Because changing behavior is hard work. If we're going to change the body, we must change the mind. As research has shown, the best results come one step—one tiny step—at a time. And it all starts in the mind.

I tell my patients to gently introduce small changes into their lives. These are called "points of choice." Make a small decision and follow that decision devotedly. Don't try to change everything at once. That way, you're much more likely to turn good intentions into everyday routine.

You may choose to start with weight management and nutritional issues. For example, if you drink 2 percent milk, drop down to 1 percent, or even mix them together for a week or so until your palate gets used to the lower fat content. Eventually, weeks later, start dropping down to skim (fat-free). Another technique is to try a different brand of milk, especially organic milk with a lower fat content. Sometimes the change in brand gives you a whole new flavor.

Or you may begin with short bouts of physical activity (note that I didn't use the "E" word—*exercise*). Spring is always a good time to start outdoor activities. If you live where you can plant a garden, with flowers or vegetables, the activity involved in schlepping dirt, raking, digging, and watering every day counts as exercise. No need to run out and join a gym, pay for six months in advance because they gave you a "good deal," think up a great excuse every day not to go, and then feel guilty. Exercise can start and stay at home. It's free.

If your issue is stress, perhaps you just need to take time to meditate, even 10 minutes a day, and that could mean simply sitting down and reading a book that has nothing to do with work or mantras or maharishis. Our technology is killing us. We need to unplug, we need to have zero screen time, we need to be off the grid periodically, or we will not go the distance.

You have many of these "points of choice" every day: at home (in deciding what to make for a meal, choosing one cookie instead of two, even determining when to go to bed), at the grocery store (what to put into your grocery cart, reading and comparing food labels), at work (taming your stressful schedule, slotting time for a workout, making choices from a vending machine), in a restaurant (ordering a meal, splitting the entrée with a friend), in your car (choosing to walk or bike instead, wearing a seat belt—okay, that's not negotiable, and neither is staying away from the cell phone while driving).

Pick just one thing to address today. Just one. If you become aware of these points of choice, you can then start changing your habits for good.

Changing for Good

Psychologists say our behavior determines our health. But knowing what to do doesn't always mean you'll do it. It's the old "I know I should exercise but ..." rationalization.

Change is a good thing, but only if you're ready. So how can you identify your readiness to change? James O. Prochaska, Ph.D., a behavioral-change guru, and his colleagues at the University of Rhode Island's Cancer Prevention Research Center identified these stages of behavior change:

- Precontemplation
- Contemplation
- Preparation
- Action
- Maintenance
- Termination

"If you're not ready, it's like trying to make a garden without preparing the soil," Dr. Prochaska says.

Precontemplation

This is known as the how-you-gonna-get-'em-up-off-the-couch stage. If you're in the precontemplation stage, you're not even thinking about making a change in your life. You might be thinking any or all of the following:

- I'll never be able to lose weight, even 10 pounds, so why bother? (Feeling hopeless.)
- I can't quit smoking. I've tried many times before; nothing works. (Feeling helpless.)
- Exercise is not a high priority for me; I don't have time right now anyway. (Denying there is a problem.)
- I can quit smoking anytime, but not right now. (Again, denying there is a problem.)

To move forward from precontemplation is a huge step in the behavior change process. *Many people never move forward from this stage.*

Your wife nagging you to stop smoking probably won't work, and she knows it. But a major life event may suddenly launch your efforts to adopt healthier behaviors. The birth of a child or grandchild can jar your thinking.

I know a husband and wife who stopped smoking on the birth of their first grandchild, but they agreed that they would resume smoking when they were 80. The thought that they would smoke again was enough to help them stop. They made the leap from precontemplation right into the action stage, and they never slipped back. So far, they've celebrated the granddaughter's high school graduation, attended her college graduation, and danced at her wedding. The age of 80 came and went. Of course, neither one is even considering smoking again. But it was the thought that counted, and it jump-started their behavior change.

The nurses who staff a health system's tobacco quit lines assist people who want to stop smoking. They know that many smokers who call aren't ready to quit yet, but some smoker's spouse may have nagged enough to get him or her to make the call. That's why the nurses use a 45-minute assessment questionnaire to screen the serious quitters. By asking pointed questions about smoking habits, the nurses can tell who is moving toward quitting and the next step, and who is stuck in precontemplation. In fact, those who are not really ready are not entered into the program; instead, they are sent information and phoned in a month for another assessment of their readiness to change.

By using these stages of change, the nurses running these quit lines have an admirable 40 percent quit rate, which is far higher than most stop-smoking programs can claim. These nurses know which smokers will be successful simply by assessing their attitude toward quitting.

Admittedly, we doctors haven't done the best job of helping our patients who are stuck in precontemplation. We simply don't have time to provide the kind of lifestyle advice patients need to make a thoughtful decision. But even 18 minutes of doctorly advice on exercise, for example, can make a world of difference.

Researchers at the Cooper Institute for Aerobics Research and at 11 medical clinics found out that a little friendly advice from the doctor coupled with health education, such as a newsletter, a pedometer, and even a few phone calls, can make big differences in getting inactive adults out of the La-Z-Boy and into activity.

The study, sponsored by the National Heart, Lung, and Blood Institute and published in the *Journal of the American Medical Association (JAMA)*, involved inactive men and women, ages 35 to 75; one-third of those studied were minorities. Although none had apparent heart disease, about 85 percent had risk factors, such as being overweight or obese; having high blood pressure or high cholesterol, or both; having diabetes; and being smokers.

The surprising result is that *all the interventions—from 18 minutes of advice to hours of counseling—resulted in similar gains in women's and men's physical activity.* Researchers were stunned to find that a little help yields important improvement (as measured in cardiovascular fitness testing before, during, and after). This tells me that people do listen to their doctors, but we need to free doctors up to provide advice in the exam room, and we need to encourage them to do so.

Sometimes surviving a critical illness, such as a heart attack or stroke, or receiving a scary diagnosis is, unfortunately, another way I see patients move from precontemplation into active behavior change—simply because they have to if they want to live. We all know friends who quit smoking after a scare with severe pneumonia leading to worry about lung cancer. Or the hard-driving executive who survives the heart attack and becomes a model of wellness.

It sure doesn't hurt if your doctor brings up the subject of your smoking or your weight or your lack of physical activity. While some doctors may feel their patients don't want to hear more harping on the subject, the research I just discussed shows exactly the opposite. Patients are receptive to lifestyle counseling from their primary care doctors, and they attribute behavior change to "the doctor said ... ," according to a study that asked patients how they felt about their doctor visits and what their doctors said.

Maybe that exam-room nudge is all you need. Knowledge is powerful medicine. It moves us from not even thinking about changing our behavior to actually trying on the behavior to see if it fits—and then moving into the next stage of behavior change.

Contemplation

When you're in the contemplation stage, you're waiting for that magic moment—you say you want to change (stop smoking, lose weight, wear sunscreen, cut back on alcohol use, for examples), and you're thinking seriously about it. But you haven't taken the leap forward into actually doing it.

At this point, you struggle with yourself. You weigh the pros and cons and hope the pros win. You recognize, for example, that if you get up from the dinner table and walk around the block, you can fit some exercise into your day. You visualize yourself going to a restaurant and ordering the lower-fat meal. You see yourself in your life as you practice the health behavior you wish to change.

How do you get to that magic moment? If we only knew. What motivates you? That's the critical piece of information in this puzzle. Is it wearing a size 10 again? Or fitting into the suit you wore when you were married? Saving the money you would have spent on cigarettes? Whatever it is, you must see yourself being successful. That will move you into the next stage of change.

Preparation

Nearly there. You have decided to take action within the next 30 days. You're beyond thinking about it; you're ready to change. You're committed to change. At this point, you may even have an action plan. Smokers might set a quit date. Future exercisers may tour a nearby gym or check out a walking trail or buy sturdy walking shoes.

You've thought about the behavior change, you see yourself doing it, and now you're ready to take action.

Action

This is it. You are practicing the behavior change you thought about and prepared for. You're cutting back your portion sizes. Or you've stopped smoking. Maybe you check your blood sugar as often as your doctor suggested. You're participating in the warm-water therapy sessions to ease the pain of your fibromyalgia. Whatever action you have adopted, congratulations!

Success is its own reward. You may find yourself falling back into your old ways, but one Häagen-Dazs ice cream doesn't doom your efforts to lose weight. You'll cut calories at your next meal. Even a smoking relapse isn't complete failure. You learned from the quitting experience, and you may slip back one step before moving ahead again. Many people find themselves moving from the action stage back to preparation but not often back to contemplation.

Maintenance

Once you have incorporated the change into your life, you enter the maintenance stage. Everything isn't easy sailing, though. You continue to work at practicing your new behavior, but it's not a struggle anymore. You know what might set you back (a particularly delicious-looking dessert or a stressful life event), but you're wary of these triggers, and you know how to cope and keep up your vigilance. You've come a long way. Some people simply remain in this stage.

Termination

Temptation no longer rears its head in the termination stage. No way will you ever smoke again. Fried food? Forget it. One drink and that's it. Taking your blood pressure medicine is the first thing you do every day. You buckle up without thinking about it. You're a regular in the Monday and Thursday aerobics class.

Whatever change you contemplated, prepared for, practiced, and took action to do, now that behavior is as automatic as brushing your teeth. This is the final step in true behavior change.

My Lifestyle Rx

Change doesn't come easy. It's not always lasting. But it's definitely worth a try.

What are your targets? What do you want to change? Just reading this book may take you from precontemplation into higher stages of behavior change in one or more areas. Just the fact that you're reading about health issues tells me you are certainly contemplating change somewhere in your life.

We'll look at each of the major lifestyle areas for behavior change in greater depth, and I'll give you my best thinking on what you can do to break down the barriers that are keeping you from adopting healthier habits and living a healthier life. You can start by taking tiny steps and moving through the stages of change, because the best part about taking small steps is that they add up to giant steps over time.

But, first, I'm going to take you into the exam room. You will learn how to talk so your doctor will listen, and I'll explain the lessons I never learned in medical school. You'll become an empowered patient. (And, for right now, you don't even have to take off your clothes or sit on an examination table!)

3

How to Talk
So Your Doctor Will Listen

No one teaches doctors to listen.
But patients deserve to be heard.

What's the one question your doctor should always ask you, but rarely ever does?

If your doctor spends time with you, talking about your health, consider yourself lucky. Some skilled clinicians can home in on your major health concerns in just a few minutes. But you need to talk to your doctor, face-to-face, with your clothes on—and your doctor needs to listen. Here's why.

In conducting a thorough head-to-toe exam, your doctor should start first by asking you this key question: *How are you feeling?* or *How are things going?* Take that question very seriously. The doctor is looking for any change in your state of good health, and really wants to know, so answer honestly. Always mention the big things, such as weight gain or loss, headaches in the morning or that awaken you from sleep, difficulty swallowing, shortness of breath, and the like. Your doctor should ask you if you have abdominal pain, problems with urination (can't go, go all the time), lumps and bumps, a sore that doesn't heal, a chronic cough.

If you're a new patient, many doctors will ask you to fill out a comprehensive questionnaire that contains a wide range of questions—often as you wait in the waiting room. If your doctor doesn't run through the entire checklist with you during your regular physical exam, insist on filling one out every time anyway. It just might uncover some health issues you need to bring up during your exam.

If right now you're thinking that your doctor doesn't ask you any questions like this, then maybe you need to find a doctor who does—or work with the doctor you see now by becoming an empowered, proactive patient. Let's look at what you should expect from your doctor and how you can make that encounter more productive.

Why People Don't Go to the Doctor, and Why They Should

I'm assuming, of course, that you make regular appointments for age-appropriate screening tests. We all know about the 90-year-old lady who seems to be the picture of health and has never been to a doctor "in her life"—or at least since her children were born decades earlier, and even then she didn't need him (yes, they were all men when she was a young woman). But that's not typical or wise.

Other people, mostly men, feel it's a sign of weakness to go to a doctor, so men avoid doctors like the plague, even if they think they have the plague. The prevalence of walk-in, no-waiting clinics has made time in front of an M.D. a little easier and faster, but Americans still practice procrastination when it comes to facing anything medical.

It's no mystery why people don't go to the doctor. Do these excuses sound familiar?

- I'm too busy.
- I'm okay. I know what's going on. I read about it on the Internet.
- I tried home care (or a supplement or an alternative medicine practitioner), and it seems to be working.
- I don't want the doctor to tell me to stop smoking and drinking.
- The doctor can't help me.
- I'm afraid of needles.

- I don't want to wait.
- I can't afford it. It's not covered by my insurance.
- I don't want to know.
- I don't have a doctor.
- I'm really okay. I don't need any of this medical stuff.

And of course there's the old familiar, "I didn't think my symptoms were bad enough to need a doctor."

A group of patients was interviewed for a study published in the *British Medical Journal*. Many felt their symptoms weren't severe enough to seek medical care, although these people were eventually diagnosed with heart attacks! They had been confused about whether they were having chest pain or indigestion, and they had hoped their discomfort would go away. If the symptoms appeared on weekends or at night, these unaware heart attack patients said they were especially reluctant to seek help during these off-hours.

So if people are not seeking medical attention for such critical, life-threatening conditions as heart attacks, they certainly are not scheduling regular appointments for basic medical screening, and they will continue to find excuses not to.

I recently read about a large managed care group, and I won't mention the name, that gave bonuses to the telephone-service representatives in their call centers if they reduced the time they spent talking with patients who were calling to schedule doctors' appointments. In addition, the phone reps were financially rewarded if they kept the number of callers actually scheduling appointments low—between 15 and 35 percent.

Frankly, I had to read the article twice because I simply could not believe that a medical organization was rushing people through the appointment process and, on top of that, discouraging their clients from seeing a doctor. We know it's sometimes quite difficult to pick up the phone and make that call in the first place. You surely don't need more barriers standing between you and medical care. Happily, however, the medical group dropped the practice.

You don't have to give your medical history or even discuss why you wish to see the doctor with the person who answers the phone at the doctor's office. Your goal is to make an appointment. That's it.

Don't let the scheduler discourage you from coming in. And if your need is urgent, say so; they'll work you in.

If you are not satisfied with that interaction, ask to speak to the doctor's nurse, who can talk with you, make an immediate assessment, or phone you back within a matter of a few hours. They do this all the time. It's part of their job as ringmaster of the doctor's schedule. Generally, the person answering the phone is a scheduler, not a medically trained staff member. Make your wishes known or ask to speak with a higher-level staff member.

Get Your 16 Minutes' Worth

The average doctor visit ranges from just 13 to 16 minutes; sometimes 20. You can make those precious minutes productive, or you can sit there and waste "your" time while the doctor never gets around to the "real" reason you showed up in the office. It's proven that many patients (mostly men) finally get around to mentioning the blood in the stool, or the chest pain, when the doctor has his or her hand on the exam room doorknob and is about to exit.

To get your 16 minutes' worth, try to be the first patient in the morning. The doctor is fresher and might be more on schedule than later in the day. Chances are you'll get more of the doctor's time. You don't want to be scheduled at 11:30, just before lunch. You're definitely not going to get in on time. Another option is to be the first appointment after lunch. Frankly, the best time for a physical exam is the day after Thanksgiving, the week after Christmas, or around other holidays; nobody wants to see a doc at holiday time. That's when most people are not focused on their health, and the waiting rooms are nearly empty.

Bring with you everything you think the doctor may need. In fact, send medical records ahead, but also bring your records (a three-ring binder, a CD of imaging, X-rays) especially if you're seeing a new doctor. And I'll discuss medical records in much more detail later in this chapter because they really are vital—you need to keep your own records.

What are your expectations when you visit the doctor? Studies often ask patients in the waiting room what they want from their visit to a general practitioner. After the appointment, the researchers then ask whether the patients' expectations were met. Most patients wanted the doctor to listen to them and then talk about their concerns. They felt this partnership would result in a mutual agreement about treatment. Patients also wanted the doctors to discuss how to stay healthy and reduce their risks for illness.

Interestingly, studies are finding that when doctors take the time to have a dialogue about a condition, patients don't want (or need) prescription medication. How quickly some doctors dash off a prescription, tear it off the pad, and send the patient packing to the pharmacy, when in fact most patients don't want a prescription at all. They might want a prescription for a healthier life, but they don't necessarily want drugs.

If you want to increase your chances of working with a doctor who will spend more time with you, choose a female physician. On average, studies find they listen more, and their appointment times last longer.

Unsaid but not forgotten

"Silence is not always golden," according to University of California–Davis researchers in the *Archives of Internal Medicine,* and what is left unsaid in the exam room is not necessarily forgotten by the patient. This research found that 9 percent of patients had something they wanted to ask their physicians but did not. Subsequently, they reported less improvement in their symptoms. Patients wanted to ask for more medical information, for a physical exam, for a diagnostic test or procedure, new medications, or referral to a specialist—but they didn't ask.

Whose fault is that?

Whether you, like these patients, feel intimidated or simply forget to ask, there is a way to make sure that your questions will be addressed. I suggest you mail, fax, or e-mail your doctor a brief note a day or two ahead of your scheduled appointment in order to alert the doctor about the major things you are concerned about. Say this: *Dear Dr. Jones, I am looking forward to our appointment on Tuesday. I'm especially concerned about a nagging cough and some pain in my abdomen.* This clues the doctor in to what is going on.

Contrary to what many people do, I advise you not to bring a long laundry list of health concerns, because you'll get sidetracked on whether you need to take fish oil, and then you will not get to the much more important concern about morning headaches. But do bring a list of all medications you are taking, their dosages and frequency, who prescribed each and why, and include herbals, supplements, and vitamins you buy for yourself without a prescription.

Who teaches doctors to listen?

Actually, no one teaches doctors to listen. Not in medical school. Medical students and residents receive little effective training in the human interactions of their craft, according to a consensus of expert teachers reported in *JAMA*. Humanism in medicine can be taught only at the bedside. That's where I have polished my skills, and I teach others in my role as professor at the Mayo Medical School.

Some medical schools teach interviewing skills. Our students role-play with each other and with medical school faculty and with trained actors. Valuable skills are taught, such as introducing yourself to the patient and making eye contact. A new study in the *Journal of Participatory Medicine* observed that doctors who make a lot of eye contact are viewed as more likable and empathetic by patients. Much of the nonverbal social communication, such as handshakes or a pat on the back, are an important link in the doctor-patient relationship.

We want our doctors to use language patients can understand. It's one thing to dictate a diagnosis of hypercholesterolemia for the patient's chart, but that means nothing to the patient until the doctor explains that it is the clinical term for high cholesterol. And then takes it further by explaining what cholesterol is and how it affects the heart and risk for stroke.

If your doctor uses terms you don't understand, by all means, stop and ask, "What are you saying?" or "Can you help me understand what that means to me?"

We on the medical school faculty are trying to convey to our students that the doctor-patient relationship should be a partnership.

We see our patients in tiny exam rooms and offices. This is an environment where patients are not always comfortable. Granted we are not all excellent communicators, but this face-to-face encounter clearly is an interaction that we can teach our medical students to handle well. Many medical schools now have videos of experienced clinicians evaluating patients, and also residents, interns, and medical students interviewing patients. The students can learn what works, and what does not work, and how to home in on a patient's concerns.

Role-modeling has an enormous impact in medical education. We typically mirror our mentors. If they do procedures a certain way, their students naturally follow suit. In past generations, some of our mentors were not effective communicators, and those skills were passed on to the next generation. However, it is no longer "business as usual," and patients should not tolerate poor communication from their primary caregivers.

It's our job to help our patients talk about what concerns them during an exam-room interaction. Because of embarrassment, patients may be reluctant to talk about their inability to achieve an orgasm or an erection, and they may visit the doctor under the pretext of having a "cough" or "feeling tired." A good medical "listener" will help the patient get to the important reason for having come to see the doctor—and will do so long before attempting to leave the room.

We physicians need to be detectives. Patients may not always tell us what we need to know. Therefore, we take clues from the patient's eye contact, body language, and voice inflection. Other indicators we can observe and even smell will give us additional clues.

If a patient complains of a cough, for example, and admits to being a heavy smoker, the astute clinician may put two and two together and investigate the cough more thoroughly. A pack of cigarettes in the patient's pocket is another sign, as is a strong smell of cigarette smoke. Suspecting something more serious than a simple cough, the careful doctor may order appropriate tests, such as a CT scan. On the other hand, the busy, hassled doctor with mediocre observation and interviewing skills may miss this opportunity to detect an important condition and send the patient away with a prescription for a cough medication.

What makes patients happy?

Go into your exam with a clear understanding of your concerns. What is the symptom? You don't have to know all the medical terms. Just tell the doctor exactly what's going on. It is helpful to write down these cues because, under the pressure of time and with the stress of being in a medical environment, patients sometimes forget these details.

Patients need the support and encouragement of family members and friends. If you bring someone to your exam with you, please make it clear that they should observe but not insert their own prejudices and concerns. After all, they are not the patient. Your needs come first. The patient should sit next to the doctor, and there should not be a family member between the patient and the doctor. This is a symbolic intrusion. This is your time.

It is also important for the doctor to end the interview with the following statement: "Are there any other concerns? Any further issues? What did we not touch on?" This signals you that the medical assessment is coming to a close. Take one of the doctor's business cards at the front desk if the doctor has not offered you one.

Did you ever try to have a conversation with someone who simply wasn't listening? It's difficult at best. Both verbal and nonverbal cues tip you off to problems in communication or lack of it. During office visits, doctors can either engage you with good listening and communication skills or completely turn you off, shuffling through a paper file, fiddling with the computer mouse, allowing staff to knock and interrupt, taking phone calls.

Researchers from the University of North Carolina, writing in the *Journal of the American Board of Family Practice*, looked at ways doctors can improve communication with their patients and whether those techniques improved patient outcomes.

Their findings showed that satisfied patients remembered what the doctor said, were pleased with the office visit, intended to comply with the treatment, and felt trust in the doctor. In the long term, these patients had improved quality of life. So what did these doctors do to make their patients happy?

The doctors showed empathy and gave reassurance and support. The visits tended to be longer, and the doctors spent more time taking the patient's medical history and explaining treatment options. They used humor and focused on the patient's feelings and emotions. The successful doctors with happy patients also spent time on health education. They shared information in a friendly way and summarized the discussion.

Nonverbally, the better communicators were perceived to show interest in the patient by nodding their heads and leaning forward—all outward signs of attention. They uncrossed their legs and arms to show with their body language that they were listening.

Not magic. Simple as that.

The expert listener typically faces the patient, makes solid eye contact, and is not distracted by pagers, beepers, knocks on the door, or noises from the waiting room. This is your time, and it should not be diluted by distractions. I personally bristle when I am with a physician (when I am the patient), and the physician answers the pager or picks up the telephone.

Expect your doctor to listen, to lean forward with an attentive posture, and, occasionally, to write down comments and concerns. Your doctor should *not* be preoccupied with entering information into electronic devices, especially if he or she is not facing you.

The doctor will "e" you now

Today's medical offices are transitioning to electronic medical record keeping. You may see nurses and doctors referring to a tablet, laptop, or desktop computer screen for reviewing your records or reciting a list of your medications. Fine. Or for looking up your previous glucose test results. Also fine. Or for checking to see if you have had a tetanus booster in the last 10 years. Once again, fine. All these are important functions for electronic medical records.

Yet as efficient as this technology is, it can also create a barrier between you and your doctor. Even physicians say the systems are cumbersome. We don't like doing anything that prevents us from providing quality care. Docs often see maintaining the electronic record as doing clerical work, according to a RAND study.

It's reasonable to say something like this: "I know you will be recording my information electronically, but could you just listen to me before turning to the computer?"

The use of the electronic medical record has now become embedded into the practice of medicine for every practitioner, and while it provides some efficiencies, it also can provide some challenges. Let me explain.

Patients treated at many medical centers can easily access their medical records, including laboratory data; they can see the results of images (such as PET scans) and hear the narration of the physician. The Veterans Administration medical system also allows patients to view lab results online. It is important for patients to understand their health conditions, but this access can provide some painful misunderstandings.

Here's an example. For many blood tests there is a range of normal. Sodium in the blood, for example, depending on the laboratory method, can have a range of 134 to 142. Yet, in the vast majority of patients, an elevation of the sodium to 143 or 144 is clinically irrelevant and has no impact on health and well-being.

I can recall a patient who contacted her provider late in the evening when she accessed her records and was terrified at this minor blip in her laboratory values. The number was of no significance whatsoever, and the patient was reassured that this was okay.

Let me share with you another example, this one far more painful. A gentleman in his 40s had the removal of a serious liver cancer and was doing fine. One of his liver blood studies was slightly abnormal, and this was explained to the patient. The patient went home, performed a Google search on this minor abnormality, and learned that it could represent bone cancer. This was not the case in this particular patient. There was another reason for the elevation, but the patient spent a miserable weekend thinking that the cancer from the liver had spread to his bone.

So the lesson is clear. Just as we might seek the input of credentialed financial professionals and accountants to sort out the nuances of our 401(k) plans, we also need the insight and judgment of the health care community in the interpretation of laboratory studies and diagnostic tests.

Germophobia or common sense?

I don't have the science on this, but consider the number of germs circulating in a doctor's waiting room and exam rooms. The odds are that people have been coming and going all day in these spaces. Children sneeze and don't cover their mouths. Adults cough and don't cover their mouths either. Germs tag along on any hard surface, and they can live there for days until picked up by another unsuspecting hand. We do know all this for a certainty.

In the home, the germiest surfaces are actually your kitchen sink and refrigerator handle. You're almost better off eating in the bathroom. Cell phones and computer keyboards are as bad as the kitchen sink, if not worse. And in public settings, door handles, elevator buttons, ATM buttons, and grocery carts are cesspools for germs. But I digress.

Even though germs are everywhere in our environment, chances are you may encounter them in any medical setting. Doctors' stethoscopes have been culprits studied as carrying germs from patient to patient.

It makes sense to be extra careful. Wash and sanitize your hands often in a medical setting. And everywhere else too, especially during flu season.

Another practice by doctors that is important is the formal washing of the hands. This signifies that the physical exam is about to begin. It is also a gesture of respect for the patient—not to mention hygienically appropriate. Even though you may be uncomfortable saying this, it's perfectly acceptable to say, "Doctor, I would appreciate your washing your hands before you examine me."

You may see providers wave their hands under a hand sanitizer instead of performing a formal soap-and-water washing. They may even don gloves. Fine. The sanitizers are acceptable ways to cleanse hands, and the alcohol-based solutions eliminate 99.9 percent of germs within a minute. Many of my colleagues carry hand sanitizers in their pockets or on their belts. This is a wise choice, especially in public places. You are especially at risk in hospitals and doctors' offices—and so are we doctors.

Male or female doctor? Does it matter?

The decision to select a male or female physician is a personal one. In general, most studies suggest that women are more comfortable with female physicians, and that is certainly understandable. One of my best friends is a prominent oncologist, and his primary health care provider is a woman. He finds that she listens to him, is sensitive to his concerns, and thoroughly assesses his condition.

Gender does make a difference, though. Female primary care doctors tend to spend more time with their patients (two minutes more, on average) and engage in more active partnership communication than male physicians, according to a study in *JAMA*. Researchers at Johns Hopkins looked at studies comparing male and female doctors for the past 30 years. At the beginning of this chapter, I introduced the one question doctors should always ask but rarely do: *How are you feeling?* The female doctors, according to research, engage in more emotional discussion around that question, although both male and female doctors delivered similar medical information.

What role does race play? It turns out that you're more likely to be satisfied with your doctor if you and the doctor are the same race, according to research also at Johns Hopkins and published in the *Journal of Health and Social Behavior*. The researchers speculated that patients, when they have a choice, will choose doctors of the same race because they are more likely to trust and feel greater comfort with such doctors. There may be an intrinsic sense of connection. Already you can see we will need many more doctors from various racial and ethnic groups to serve our growing diverse populations.

If it's important to be seen by a doctor of your own race, then by all means factor that into your selection process. A satisfied patient is much more likely to comply with treatment, to keep follow-up appointments, and, although doctors won't admit it, less likely to bring a malpractice suit in the event of a problem or bad medical outcome.

This begs the question: What makes a good doctor? What qualities are you looking for in choosing a doctor? Qualities of empathy and sensitive communication are far more important than gender or race.

The bottom line is that patients, no matter their gender or race or their doctor's gender or race, want to be listened to. In effect, the patient is saying, "Make me feel important. Acknowledge my concerns. Don't write me off."

If the chemistry between you and your doctor is not positive, if the energy or karma is not in sync, you certainly have the right to request and seek another physician. This can be done very discreetly, is a common practice, and is clearly your right.

Inside the Exam Room (Behind the Curtain)

Imagine you're sitting in the exam room, the doctor comes in, says hello, and asks how to help. Imagine you begin speaking and talk until you are finished. The doctor doesn't interrupt. How long do you think most patients will talk if they are not interrupted?

Researchers reporting on a study in the *British Medical Journal* tried just that. Doctors were asked to time their patients, using a hidden stopwatch, and not interrupt until the patient said something like, "What do you think, doctor?"

The average talk time was just 92 seconds, and most patients (78%) finished within 2 minutes. Older patients tended to talk longer. The doctors felt that their patients were providing important information and did not feel the need to interrupt. But that was a forced study.

In actual practice, doctors interrupt in about 20 seconds.

Unless you talk fast, it is absolutely crucial that you have the opportunity to voice your concerns without being shortchanged by the physician jumping in. If the physician interrupts you, I think it is appropriate to say, "Doctor, I appreciate your jumping in, but please let me finish this thought." This is a reasonable gesture to clearly get your points out.

Should you make and take a list with you? Only a short one, unless you already sent your doctor a note a few days before your appointment, as recommended earlier in this chapter. Your doctor will appreciate it if you are organized. There are a few other things you might consider taking with you: a pen and paper, even a friend. Please write down what the doctor says. It's perfectly acceptable, and I encourage it. Better yet, your friend can take notes while you engage in a dialogue with the doctor. Of course, this works best if you are comfortable bringing your spouse or sister or caring friend, but many people are not at ease with this.

The downside is that a well-meaning family member or friend can interfere with the doctor-patient relationship by attempting to show off newly found medical knowledge from the Internet or inserting his or her own medical story into the conversation. But the upside is that you will remember (together) what the doctor said—and understand it.

Often, I see patients accompanied by many family members. In general, I'm seeing my patients at a clearly difficult time. They usually have a serious, life-threatening illness, and their support group is an essential part of their treatment. Everyone has to be on board, and the patient has called upon them to help in the decision making.

Routine exams, however, usually can be handled alone, but feel free to take notes and to ask the doctor to repeat information you didn't hear or don't understand. Some practical and reasonable questions may be these:

- What is my diagnosis? What's going on with me?
- What treatment do you suggest? What are my options?
- What should I be doing now to manage this condition?
- Where can I find out more about my condition?
- What's the reasonable expected track record of my condition? Where do you think my condition will be in three to six months?

If you are given a prescription, it's sensible to ask these questions:

- What is this medication? What symptoms does it treat?
- How much do I take? When and how do I take it?
- What are the possible side effects?
- How will I know if it is working?
- Does this drug interact with any other medications, vitamins, supplements, or herbals I am taking?
- What should I do if I forget to take it?
- How much does it cost? (If too much, is there a generic or an appropriate substitute?)

Your pharmacist can respond to some of these questions about medication, but the best person to ask first is your doctor. Don't wait until you're home from the pharmacy to read the label or printout that comes with your prescription. If you have questions, or you can't remember what the doctor said, call the doctor's office. The doctor's nurse should be able to get answers and get back to you.

What patients want (and need) to hear

Whatever brings you inside a doctor's exam room, you know what you want to hear from the doctor, and if you don't get answers, reassurance, and education from your physician, you will not think you have had a successful medical interaction. Never mind that you may not comply with treatment or that you might have to call the doctor later if your condition gets worse.

One concerned mother took her son to a dermatologist to find out about some white spots on his face. From start to finish, the entire interaction took less than one minute, and during that time, the doctor said, "Don't worry, Mom," four times.

He walked into the exam room, glanced at the child, dashed off a prescription, stuck it in her hand, and dashed out the door, leaving a frustrated mother with a host of unanswered questions, not to mention an impatient five-year-old sporting white spots on his face.

Sound familiar?

The problem may have been trivial, but the doctor should not have treated it as such. I can guarantee you that the mother may not seek help for another alarming rash that could be more serious. And she certainly won't return to this doctor for treatment ever again.

What the mother needed to hear was this: "Nothing serious, it's just a *blah blah blah,* and it will go away on its own in a week or two. If not, call me. You can put this cream on it to help it go away faster. We're not sure why things like this appear, but it's not contagious."

With this ideal answer, the doctor could have anticipated and answered questions, and still been out the door in a couple of minutes. "Don't worry" was a poor substitution for solid information. And I don't care how much of a hurry the doctor is in, how many calls are on hold, and how many patients are backed up sitting in little exam rooms or in the waiting room, we doctors owe you our time and attention—that's our job. First and foremost, you're the patient. You can decide if you want to worry. The point of honest answers to your questions is to allay your fears.

Some patients go to the doctor with the expectation that they will be given a prescription and everything will be just fine—as if drugs could fix just about anything. Research shows that patients who expected medication were nearly three times more likely to receive a prescription. When the doctor *thought* the patient expected medication, the patient was 10 times more likely to receive it.

That's why patients are walking out of clinics everywhere with prescriptions for antibiotics when what they have is a viral infection or common cold that a little chicken soup could help (but that's discussed in another chapter). Antibiotic resistance is a growing concern simply because patients are asking for these potent medications, expecting a prescription, and doctors are complying even when they know a patient won't be helped by it—just because doctors are afraid to send a patient out the door empty-handed. How about filling their minds with information? After all, knowledge is powerful medicine.

Asking for specific medications is a concern because we are seeing an increase in what is called direct-to-consumer drug advertising on TV, in print media, and online. Compelling ads for "the pill that's ready when you are" or for the "purple pill" are driving you to ask your doctor specifically for them. I've seen prescription fulfillment numbers as high as 30 percent, indicating that doctors are giving patients the medications they are asking for—whether those meds are appropriate or not. That's the downside.

On the upside (and I do refer here to erectile dysfunction medications), patients motivated by TV commercials can become more active in their treatment. If a news item or drug commercial opens a dialogue between you and your doctor, so much the better. A wise practitioner will seize that teachable moment to discuss your complete health picture and, I hope, take time to explore all your options. Requests for Viagra got men into doctors' offices in record numbers. With such motivated patients, smart doctors are taking blood pressures and getting cholesterol levels too. And dispensing prescriptions for Viagra and other medications, if appropriate.

Patients listen when doctors prescribe a healthy lifestyle

Often lost in the doctor-patient dialogue are matters of lifestyle choice. The whole notion of shared decision making is forgotten in that 16-minute encounter. Other patients are waiting. The phones are ringing. Time is ticking away. Who has time to talk about quitting smoking or losing weight? Patient-centered care is a key concept here.

But it's critical for doctors to take time and make time to counsel you on lifestyle issues, whether you are there for that type of information or not. Why? Simply because people trust the doctor's advice more than any other source, and also because a doctor's advice changes behavior.

How do I know this? The U.S. Preventive Services Task Force said that personalized advice from a doctor about breaking bad habits or adopting a healthier lifestyle enhances the patient's motivation to change, which may be that extra push from precontemplation or not even thinking about changing (discussed in the previous chapter on behavior change) into contemplation (thinking about change) and action stages (actually making lifestyle changes).

Because half of the top 10 causes of death are linked to behaviors, such as smoking, inactivity, poor diet, alcohol misuse, and obesity, the federal task force has suggested that doctors may even convey health messages phrased like this: "As your physician, I feel I should tell you …" as a subtle yet powerful way of engaging you, the patient, in shared decision making.

Can these messages make a difference? Researchers at the University of Wisconsin–Madison wanted to know what would happen if doctors talked to their patients for a few minutes about drinking habits. Alcohol contributes to liver disease, cancer, and problems with developing fetuses in pregnant women, and it's a leading cause of domestic violence, child abuse, accidents, and injury. A worthy target for intervention.

Patients aged 18 to 65 who were seeing doctors on routine visits were given a screening questionnaire to look at their at-risk alcohol behaviors. Those who screened positive—meaning they had risky alcohol behaviors, such as drinking alone or drinking too much at times—were given two 15-minute face-to-face conversations with their doctors, followed by two 5-minute phone calls from a nurse.

Discussions centered on what was acceptable drinking behavior and how to monitor drinking habits.

Short-term results are always encouraging, but it's the long-term behavior change that truly makes a difference, and it did in this experiment. The study participants were followed up over a period of years. Early intervention by the family doctor made a huge difference, even four years after the doctor-patient discussion, by reducing alcohol-related illness and injury.

The bottom line is that it's cost-effective for doctors to spend a few minutes talking with new and established patients about their alcohol habits, and, as a result of such conversations, up to 20 percent of patients will significantly decrease their alcohol use. In doing so, they lower their risk for accidents and reduce their overall health care costs as well. It's also important for doctors to discuss alcohol use for another reason: If the doctor is going to prescribe any medication, the doctor needs to know what other medications the patient is taking, even Tylenol, in order to avoid serious alcohol-drug interactions.

Smokers are tough to reach. Sometimes it seems our nonsmoking messages are falling on deaf ears, but a study at Case Western Reserve University showed that smokers welcome counseling about smoking cessation from their family doctors. In fact, they are more satisfied with their physician visits if the doctors provide this type of counseling. And it's more than just "you need to stop smoking." One study showed that talking about smoking for as little as three minutes was likely to be effective.

Equally important, in my opinion, is for doctors to give advice about physical activity. The Surgeon General, along with many other groups, promotes 30 minutes of moderate activity on most days of the week. Others say 60 minutes is better, but the truth is that 70 percent of patients are underactive, and that includes children and adolescents. This decline in activity is certainly attributed to television, video games, and computers, all leading to a steep rise in obesity, type 2 diabetes (yes, in our children), colon cancer, and high blood pressure. These chronic conditions often don't appear until middle age, but they have their roots in childhood.

The family physician is perfectly positioned to provide counseling about physical activity, and a study by one of my colleagues at Mayo Clinic calls for doctors to literally jump in and "prescribe" exercise.

Only half of patients receive advice from their doctors to get moving and to increase their levels of activity. It's time for doctors to write prescriptions for a healthy life in an attempt to tear our patients away from keyboards and TV remotes, get them to walk away from the refrigerator and fast food, and encourage them to be active.

A little doctorly advice goes a long way

Here's another area in which we can do better: Most women still don't know that folic acid must be taken before pregnancy to prevent certain defects in newborns. Prevention works. Yet doctors fail to tell women of childbearing age to take a multivitamin containing folic acid to prevent birth defects if they become pregnant, according to a March of Dimes study. Patients hear and heed lifestyle messages. I hope your physician is riding the white horse of patient education.

The fact of the matter is that doctors do a poor job of providing information (in person and in written educational materials), according to researchers in the Center for Cost and Outcomes Research at the University of Washington–Seattle. Too often, medical decisions fall into a gray area where the best choice for any individual may be unclear and where reasonable people might choose differently. Common examples are certain procedures for back pain or treatment for benign (harmless) prostate problems. Which drugs to choose for treatment is another gray area where risks, benefits, and side effects need to be weighed.

These types of decisions are made daily in doctors' offices; nevertheless, many questions remain. If you are to become an empowered patient, you must go into the medical arena armed with information (or know where to get the best decision-making tools), because you simply cannot expect to get that from your doctor.

Older patients tend to defer medical decisions to the doctor (our "Greatest Generation" still thinks the doctor knows best). But that does not mean these older patients are happy with their treatment. Research in the *British Medical Journal* demonstrated that such factors as knowledge of risk, the doctor's ability to communicate, and the doctor-patient relationship are critical to informed choice. The goal is to get to informed choice yourself and not rely solely on the doctor to get you there, because the doctor simply can't. This must be a partnership, not a dictatorship; it must work for you and with you.

Is There a Doctor in the Mouse?

The lifestyle and health decisions you make can mean the difference between life and death—yours. You want the best opinions and the most current and trusted medical advice. If not at your doctor's office, then where can you find it? You can get good medical advice on the Internet, but you have to be a savvy shopper and use it to help you, not hurt you.

A patient of mine nearly died because his wife purchased what she thought was a safe "immune-system stimulant" through an unofficial alternative-medicine-type website. We were treating him for a brain tumor. She was desperate. Her husband was quite ill. She felt she was helping boost his immune system, which was so severely weakened by his condition and his treatment.

Here's what happened: He almost bled to death because of the drug interaction with the bogus substance she found online. Rather embarrassed and certainly concerned, they admitted what they had done. Using a simple search engine, I determined the ingredients of the so-called miracle cure. It was actually a blood thinner, not an "immune-system stimulant" at all.

The Internet can work for you and against you. It is a double-edged sword that can have catastrophic complications. The lesson of this story is to beware of buying medicine and medical products on the Internet, and to work with your doctor and pharmacist to check all drug interactions. Anything you put into your body should be considered in relation to everything else you put into it.

Here's another example: One of my patients developed a very rare cancer of the abdominal tissue. An unsophisticated Internet search by the desperate patient uncovered a physician in Miami who was advertising for patients. He was performing surgery on people with this condition. She was practically packed and ready to go when we discussed why that surgery was not an option for her situation.

Point, click, heal

The examples I just mentioned show how the Internet is changing the doctor-patient relationship. Our patients are turning to the Internet to access the very same medical information we doctors have been reading in journals. These patients are coming to the exam room able to begin their medical discussion at a higher level of understanding, and they are changing the way we practice.

Survey after survey still confirms that patients trust information from their doctors more than they trust information from the Internet and other sources, such as daytime TV doctor shows, books, and newspaper and magazine articles. Rather than undermining our efforts, the Internet can enhance the relationship, but doctors must help patients get to the best, most trusted places on the Internet, or they will spend precious time discussing treatments that are not appropriate for the patient sitting in front of them with a handful of computer printouts.

The solution, perhaps, is for doctors to direct patients to trusted Internet sites by providing an annotated handout, or to set up their own websites with links to approved information centers, and certainly there are plenty of well-reviewed and well-written consumer-health information sources on the Internet. The danger lies in a patient conducting a Google search and ending up in uncharted territory. Ask your doctor which websites he or she feels comfortable "prescribing."

I recommend you start any Internet search for medical or health information at a portal, mega site, or gateway, not at a general search engine such as Yahoo or Google or Bing, so you immediately get into a loop of reviewed and trusted sites.

Start searches, for example, at a major medical center's mega site such as *MayoClinic.com* or MedlinePlus at *nlm.nih.gov/medlineplus* (a site operated by the National Library of Medicine [NLM] and the National Institutes of Health [NIH]). These sites are rich with content on diseases and conditions from A to Z, and they have decision support tools to help you understand and manage chronic conditions, such as migraine or diabetes.

Other trusted sites to start a search are government portals, such as *cdc.gov, health.gov,* and *healthfinder.gov* (portals or clearinghouses from which you are directed to content-rich websites). I don't discount websites funded by educational grants from pharmaceutical companies. Sure, drug companies have a vested interest in the conditions they manufacture drugs for, but they are also robust repositories for patient information on the condition. They partner with and support nonprofit groups to get the word out. Read their information, but know that they have a self-serving interest in your using their medications.

Health-serving organizations are among the best sites to find disease-specific information. The American Heart Association (*heart.org*), American Cancer Society (*cancer.org*), American Diabetes Association (*diabetes.org*), and American Lung Association (*lung.org*) are nonprofit groups whose sole mission is to gather and convey information on a particular condition. Use them, support them, trust their information.

Ten Things to Know About Evaluating Medical Resources on the Internet

The federal government's Office on Alternative and Complementary Medicine and the Medical Library Association representing medical librarians at some of the nation's finest academic sites, among others, have developed guidelines to help you evaluate medical information on any website. Here are some highlights to guide your searches:

1. Who runs this site?

Any sound health-related website should make it easy for you to learn who is responsible for the site and its information. The sponsor should be clearly marked on every major page of the site, along with a link to the site's home page. If you can't find the sponsor easily, get outta there. If you've never heard of the sponsor, click off the site.

2. Who pays for the site?

It costs money to run a website. The source of a site's funding should be clearly stated or readily apparent. For example, web addresses ending in ".gov" denote a federal government–sponsored site. You should know how the site pays for its existence. Does it sell advertising? Is it sponsored by a drug company? Do you see banner ads or annoying pop-up ads? The source of funding can affect what content is presented, how the content is presented, and what the site owners want to accomplish on the site. On the other hand, ads aren't all bad; somebody has to pay for your free access.

3. What is the purpose of the site?

This question is related to who runs and pays for the site. An "About This Site" or "About Us" link or tab appears on many sites. If it's there, use it. The purpose of the site should be clearly stated and should help you evaluate the trustworthiness of the information.

4. Where does the information come from?

Many health/medical sites post information collected from other websites or sources. If the person or organization in charge of the site did not create the information, the original source should be clearly labeled.

5. What is the basis of the information?

In addition to identifying who wrote the material you are reading, the site should describe the evidence that the material is based on. Medical facts and figures should have references (to articles in reputable medical journals, for example, just as I have given credit in this book to studies in reputable journals). Also, opinions or advice should be clearly set apart from information that is *evidence-based* (that is, based on research results). Be skeptical about claims based on testimonials from "happy patients" or firsthand accounts of "cures."

6. How is the information selected?

Is there an editorial board? Do people with excellent professional and scientific qualifications review the material before it is posted? Sites with impressive editorial boards or medical advisory committees eagerly list credentials. Look for these links and look over the group. You want to recognize their academic affiliations and medical credentials (such as M.D.).

7. How current is the information?

Websites should be reviewed and updated on a regular basis (every two years is a good measure). It is particularly important that medical information be current. The most recent update or review date should be clearly posted (often at the end of an article). Even if the information has not changed, you want to know whether the site owners have reviewed it recently to ensure that it is still valid.

8. How does the site choose links to other sites?

Websites usually have a policy about how they establish links to other sites. Some medical sites take a conservative approach and don't link to any other sites. Some link to any site that asks, or pays, for a link. Others only link to sites that have met certain criteria.

9. What information about you does the site collect, and why?

Websites routinely track the paths visitors take through their sites in order to determine what pages are being used. However, many health sites ask you to "subscribe" or "become a member." In some cases, this may be so that they can collect a user-fee or select information for you that is relevant to your concerns. In all cases, this will give the site personal information about you. Be cautious.

Any credible health site asking for this kind of information should tell you exactly what they will and will not do with it. Many commercial sites sell "aggregate" (collected) data about their users to other companies—such as what percentage of their users are women with breast cancer, for example. In some cases, they may collect and reuse information that is "personally identifiable," such as your ZIP code, gender, and date of birth.

Be certain that you read and understand any privacy policy or similar language on the site, and don't sign up for anything that you are not sure you fully understand. Some health insurers give you a password and access to medical information sites because you are a policyholder. Take advantage of these sites, but use caution about revealing personal health information.

10. How does the site manage interactions with visitors?

There should always be a way for you to contact the site owner if you run across problems, have questions, or wish to offer feedback. If the site hosts chat rooms, forums, or other online discussion areas, it should tell visitors what the terms of using this service are. Is it moderated? If so, by whom, and why? It is always a good idea to spend time reading the discussion without joining in so that you feel comfortable with the environment before becoming a participant.

Sources: National Center for Complementary and Alternative Medicine (*nccam.nih.gov*) and the Medical Library Association's *A User's Guide to Finding and Evaluating Health Information on the Web* (*mlanet.org/resources/userguide.html*).

Keep Copies of Your Medical Records at All Times

Unheard of in the past, keeping your own set of records can be truly lifesaving. No longer is that manila file in the doctor's office the only place for everything about you, from head to toe. In fact, that manila folder has probably already been scanned, page by page, and placed into an electronic medical record.

Your health records are everywhere. Your family doctor knows when you had your last tetanus shot. The ob/gyn has information on your Pap smear, and the dermatologist has the lab report on the suspicious mole taken off your face three years ago. If you've been in the hospital, inpatient records on your hernia surgery are in their massive record rooms. The walk-in clinic has files on your previous sore throats. And the hospital's emergency department recorded your broken arm or chest pain visit.

Whatever your health status, it's absolutely essential that you gather the pieces of your medical health history and maintain your own master file of medical records.

Why? Because you need them for a number of reasons. Initially, you need to verify that all information in all your files is accurate, especially regarding information you have told the doctor. I've seen lab reports misfiled, people with similar names getting each other's physician notes, and doctors simply dictating wrong information that is transcribed inaccurately and put into your file.

But why would any of this matter?

- You may need to provide your medical history and past treatment to a new doctor. It would be senseless for a new physician to base treatment decisions on information that was inaccurately recorded or simply misfiled.
- You might be seeking specialized care from someone like me for a second opinion. We always appreciate knowing the big picture from medical records. I'll give you a lifesaving example in a minute.
- Or, let's say you are applying for life or health insurance (although preexisting conditions will no longer be considered when issuing health insurance). The prospective insurance company will ask you to sign a release so they can see your medical records. Wouldn't you want to make sure they are correct? You want to monitor what is released and to whom, according to the American Health Information Management Association.

With many different health care providers, with lab results being faxed and e-mailed, with CT scans digitally transmitted, your personal medical records can be scattered in several doctors' offices, pharmacies, and hospital system computers. And if you have more than one doctor (and most people do), assembling all the essential information in a time of crisis can be a nightmare, if not impossible.

How to gather your records

- **Start your medical record keeping right now.** At your next doctor's appointment, ask for a release form, fill it out, and sign it. Even if there's a small fee, pay it. If you have trouble getting your records, contact your state's department of health. It's your right.

- **Request a copy of everything,** including X-rays and other diagnostics, lab and other reports, and correspondence between doctors. Your doctor is required to copy and send records to you. Your doctor might hire a service that will copy the records for you (for a fee). Or you might be able to get a CD of an MRI or CT, for example, right from your doctor's office or the medical imaging facility.

- **Do this every time you see a doctor** (including specialists) or are in the hospital (pathology reports are helpful if you have surgery), and just keep building your records.

- **Track down records** from doctors you've seen in the past but no longer see. Request copies of your records. If doctors have sold their practices, retired, or moved to different health care systems, your records may take some time to locate.

- **Take key records with you** to your appointments in case your file has been "misplaced." If your doctor sees patients in different geographic locations, and paper records are still toted around in bins, they can easily become lost. Many medical offices are still transitioning into electronic medical record keeping.

Imagine the horror if you were undergoing treatment for a specific condition or tracking cholesterol, thyroid levels, or other blood results from the lab, and the doctor's records could not be found for comparison. It has happened, believe me.

I had the pleasure of treating a woman whose daughter literally saved her life. When this woman came to our clinic, she had already seen multiple doctors in many different states. The daughter had kept massive and complete three-ring binders of records during the mother's treatment for a life-threatening illness. When the patient arrived in my office, I had everything I needed to help her make a lifesaving treatment decision, knowing all the efforts and results to date—all thanks to the daughter's diligence. Otherwise, we would have wasted valuable time and made decisions about treatments that might have already been tried.

During a routine checkup, another patient looked fine, except for a spot the size of a nickel on her lung, which was revealed on a chest X-ray. We were naturally suspicious, and everything was moving toward major surgery. Somehow, we were able to find a previous physician who had given her an exam 15 years before. The chest X-ray taken then showed the same spot. Then there was no need for surgery, but we wouldn't have known that without having the earlier records for comparison.

Outcomes for you may not be so critical, but there are times when having an earlier chest X-ray or mammogram (for comparison) or laboratory test results on PSA levels, blood counts, thyroid or liver functions, or adult immunizations can make a critical difference in whether you need treatment or not.

The PSA test (a blood test to screen for prostate cancer) of a 65-year-old patient was 3.7. No problem, right? Normal is in a range between 0 and 4. Most doctors would say, "Thanks for coming; see you next year." But this patient brought along records showing that just a year earlier his PSA was 1, meaning his blood levels had increased fourfold in just a single year. So even though he was within a normal range, we arranged a biopsy, caught the cancer early, and cured it with surgery. Without his records, he would have been a year farther down the road toward advanced prostate cancer.

Another patient showed a very low hemoglobin (usually a sign of anemia), and we became concerned, until we examined the medical records and took note of his heritage. Hemoglobin is a measure of the red blood cells and their ability to carry oxygen throughout the body. His was 9, and normal is 14 to 16. Fortunately, we had available to us his medical records for the past 30 years. We all breathed a sigh of relief when we saw that he had been at 9 for years. That, coupled with the fact that he was of Italian descent, turned an abnormality into nothing. Mediterranean people can often have harmless DNA blood conditions that would produce these readings.

Until universal electronic medical record-keeping systems in the "cloud" become accessible to any doctor anywhere, with your permission, or until we each wear our medical records on a tiny computer chip inside a bracelet or necklace, we're stuck dealing with paper and electronic records scattered in every doctor's office and hospital we've ever been in (literally since birth for most of us).

Until a one-stop shop exists for all your medical records in cyberspace (it's coming), take control of your records.

Certain key medical records should be with you *at all times*. For example, keep a copy of your EKG—that's a heart tracing—in your wallet or purse if you have any heart problems. Ask your doctor for what we call a rhythm strip. It's a piece of paper about 3 feet long and 3 inches high. Simply fold it to about the size of a credit card.

Let's say you show up in the ER with chest pain, and doctors run an EKG. Let's make this interesting. You're on vacation, hundreds of miles from home. You'll get much better treatment and have a higher chance for faster and accurate treatment if doctors can compare the two readings.

If you're traveling, put this key medical record in your travel bag or briefcase. I also advise my patients who have an abnormal chest X-ray to ask us for a miniature version (about 8 by 11 inches). This might show a piece of shrapnel or a bullet that could not be removed. Some metal detectors in airports and sensitive venues will pick up these images, and you will need to explain them. You might also wear this information on a medical alert medallion or bracelet. People with pacemakers and stents often carry wallet cards detailing the device.

Ask your doctor to dictate a brief summary of your condition that can then be printed on his or her letterhead. Keep this with you (even on your smartphone along with a list of your medications). Some tech-savvy patients have their records copied and put onto a thumb drive. These devices are about the size of a tube of lipstick and can be easily accessed with any computer (especially handy if you travel).

How you can protect your privacy ... from doctors who may not even know they're violating it

Your medical information is sensitive, confidential, and just between you and your doctor. But because your medical records are no longer stored just in those familiar color-coded files in your doctor's office, your personal medical data may instantly be dispatched around the world electronically by fax or e-mail.

Unless you take proper precautions, your private medical information may not be safe. Talk with your doctor and the office staff about ways to preserve your privacy. They are required to respect your privacy, according to the federal regulation known as HIPAA (the Health Insurance Portability and Accountability Act of 1996), and you'll be asked to sign a form at every medical encounter in order to acknowledge that you were told they will preserve the confidentiality of your medical information:

In person: Discuss your privacy concerns. People most concerned about preserving privacy may have a family history of a dreaded disease they want to keep confidential, especially from employers. Most of us would want to keep confidential any issues involving sexually transmitted diseases (including HIV/AIDS), as well as pregnancy and mental illness. Find out your doctors' office policies on releasing information, and make sure you understand and agree with them. If you don't want medical information released for insurance reimbursement, don't sign a release. Pay the entire amount yourself.

By voice mail: The very fact that you are seeing a doctor is confidential. The biggest concern is that someone other than you will intercept a phone message at home or at work from your doctor's office. Sensitive medical professionals will leave only a basic message, such as, "This is Heidi calling for Mrs. Johnson. Please call me at [office number]." If you have specific wishes about where and how the medical staff may leave a message for you about test results or follow-up, or just to make an appointment, make sure the instructions get noted on your medical chart.

By e-mail: We are clearly in the age of the virtual or digital office. Without question, e-mail is not-so-subtly changing the landscape of medical practice. However, there are some major concerns. First, confidentiality. There is no such thing as a secure browser, and delicate, sensitive, and revealing medical information could wind up in the wrong hands.

If you e-mail your doctor, don't expect him or her to e-mail you back with information on medical treatment. In order to make an informed diagnosis, your doctor must examine you, and that can't be done by e-mail. Use e-mail only to set up appointments or to obtain referrals. You know how difficult it is for you to respond to multiple e-mails each day. Now imagine that load dumped on your doctor. Communicating with patients via e-mail is not reimbursed time. It's extra work that extends a doctor's already busy workday, even though such communication seems efficient and effective and improves patient satisfaction, according to a study from Weill Cornell Medical College in *Health Affairs*.

By fax: If you're expecting a fax of, say, lab results, from your doctor and you use a shared fax machine, set up a time beforehand, by phone, with the doctor's office. Confirm your incoming fax number, and babysit the fax machine until your fax arrives.

By mail: It's okay for your doctor to notify you by mail (many do) with test results or reminders about upcoming appointments, but you also have the right to request a phone call instead.

It is illegal for doctors to discuss your medical situation with anyone else, unless you have given written permission.

Reviewing and amending your records

As a patient, you have an absolute right to review your medical records—and to get copies of them. But some medical office staff may resist your request. They simply aren't used to patients asking to see their records (although such requests are becoming more common). You may ask to see the original file in your doctor's office, but you cannot take it with you. The medical record (paper or electronic) itself is the property of the doctor.

- Review your file in the doctor's office, where medical staff can explain any technical medical terminology and abbreviations. Ask the doctor to amend any incorrect information about you. Or, ask him or her to write a letter to be inserted into your file to clarify any errors. You can also insert a letter to express your own opinion. Make sure the records show your family medical history and emergency numbers, current medications, allergies, organ donor wishes, and advance directives.

- Make sure your file is complete and that all information is about you, and not about somebody with the same or similar name.
- Check and update your health insurance information, if necessary, and examine the date of all authorizations you have signed to release medical information—to whom and for what. Change or delete as appropriate.
- Ask your doctor to summarize the medical notes he or she has written after consulting with you. Many of us are part of an increasing trend of sharing clinical notes with our patients to make sure our patients are on the same page with treatment and care. We take a few minutes to go over our notes. It helps our patients feel they are part of their own care, and it also helps to ensure that they take their medications correctly.

How Healthy Is Your Family Tree?

What you don't know about your family tree could cost you your life. On the other hand, knowing your family health history can be empowering and may help you ward off medical problems. No medical record is complete without a family health history.

Does it really matter how Aunt Louise died, or whether Grandpa William had a heart condition? Yes.

We know that 10 to 15 percent of people with colon cancer have a family history that includes this disease. If one or both parents are alcoholics, we know that 25 percent of their children are at risk for becoming alcohol abusers themselves. Diabetes and high blood pressure also run in families and pose a risk.

You're not doomed to develop diseases just because they are present in your family. As I have discussed, lifestyle certainly plays a large part in disease development. With knowledge, you become more vigilant about your lifestyle habits and more diligent with early health screenings.

At your next family reunion, find out about your blood relatives' health histories—how they died, if they were overweight, and if they had any unusual or unexplained illnesses. The knowledge may save your life.

Here's a typical case: A 30-year-old woman feels just fine but notices a dimpling of one nipple. It looks different from her other breast. In most cases, if she calls it to the attention of her doctor, she'll receive a physical exam, and that might be it. Nothing to worry about. But if she mentions that her aunt is undergoing chemotherapy for breast cancer, the stakes are higher. She'd then have a mammogram, maybe an ultrasound and MRI. Her family history of breast cancer raises the index of suspicion.

It's not that conscientious doctors would miss the opportunity to find and treat an early condition, but they are busy, and overworked, and the unusual is not always on their radar screen. If you're the patient, say, "Doctor, let me tell you about my family history." That'll get the doctor's attention—and get you the proper treatment.

If Aunt Louise died under unusual circumstances and nobody is really sure how she died—and it was years ago—some clues might help you. If the story at the family reunion is that she never woke up from an operation, it could be that she was particularly vulnerable to anesthesia. And you might be too. If you're a blood relative, make sure you tell your doctor about this, and especially your anesthesiologist if you're scheduled for surgery. In these cases and with certain surgeries, you would be quite closely monitored, and you might elect to have a spinal block instead of general anesthesia. Simple, yes, but lifesaving.

Map your family health history back to your grandparents, aunts and uncles, great-aunts and -uncles, first cousins, and, of course, your parents and siblings. Important details, if available, are their gender, years of birth and death, illnesses and ongoing health conditions, ages they were when diagnosed, and their causes of death. Note lifestyle factors, such as whether they smoke(d) or are/were overweight.

You need to gather and safeguard your medical records and those of your children (until they reach adulthood). Keep your family health history with your medical records. Know as much about your family medical history as you can. Someday, those records may make the difference in lifesaving medical decisions.

My Prevention Rx

I advise you to go into the exam room fully prepared to make your all-too-brief encounter highly productive. Don't let anything deter you from your mission—not the doctor's pager or cell phone, a friend's off-track questions, weird stuff from the Internet, or trivial concerns that take time away from the big issues that brought you to the doctor in the first place. What is your mission or primary concern? You are seeing a health care professional for a specific medical question, whether this is a pain, a worry, or a routine exam.

Your doctor should give you the courtesy of letting you explain your concerns in your own words. Don't let the doctor jump in until you have had a chance to tell your story, and typically this takes only a few minutes. In other words, you are there to tell your story and to be listened to.

As clinicians, we can look at records and X-rays and test results, but we need to hear the rest of the story—and that can only be done by carefully listening to the patient.

Your obligation as a patient is to come prepared for an exchange of information. Your preparation must include knowing your medical history, and that means having medical records available. Unheard of in the past, it's now not unusual at all for someone to assemble his or her own complete medical record.

Most parents keep track of their children's immunizations faithfully because schools and camps need this information. So it's a natural extension to track a thyroid level or cholesterol or blood pressure. You want to keep track of these numbers as they increase or decrease over a period of time. From one doctor visit to another, you may move to a new city or see different doctors for various reasons. Doctors don't have a central clearinghouse for information about every person (at least not yet). Until then, the only person who can maintain continuity of care for you is *you.*

The information contained in your medical records is your property. (The actual record, paper or electronic, is the property of the doctor.) Your health information is part of you. You are entitled to copies of everything about you. You are also entitled to an explanation of your records, and it is appropriate for you to ask your health care provider for clarification when needed.

In choosing a doctor, you need to feel a positive chemistry. There needs to be the sense that the physician does care for you—the patient—and is concerned about your welfare. Obviously, complete disclosure and honesty, as well as open sharing of information, are crucial. This should be viewed as a partnership, as a relationship to safeguard your health, and, if necessary, to rally against a common foe: disease, illness, or disability.

Armed with your own medical history and a sense of empowerment to make the health care system truly care for you, you can enter any exam room prepared to talk so your doctor will listen.

4

What They Never Taught Me in Medical School

The street-smart stuff, well, we doctors learn that later—
sometimes the hard way.

Much of what we do as physicians has very little to do with what we were taught in medical school. The street-smart stuff, well, we doctors learn that later—sometimes the hard way. Let me give you some examples of what we were not taught in medical school—but stuff I know after years of practicing medicine:

- **Patients want to be acknowledged and listened to.** As I've already mentioned, that means it is not good form for your doctor to respond to interruptions, such as a phone call, knock on the door, or pager. Doctors should put these distractions off for several minutes. Doing so causes no harm. If your doctor is interrupted, make it clear that you do not want to be left in the lurch again. Emergencies are understandable, of course, but they are also rare.

- **Most patients have difficulty following treatment instructions.** Especially if you're talking with your doctor about an emotionally charged diagnosis, such as cancer or another life-changing condition, you may not remember what you discussed. Even for small office procedures, such as removal of a mole, most patients don't remember their wound-care instructions—thus jeopardizing healing.

I advise you to take notes, ask the doctor to repeat something if you didn't hear it, ask for clarification if you don't understand it, and follow up with phone calls to the doctor if you have any confusion, especially about medication. You are perfectly welcome to invite pertinent family members or close friends to sit in on the discussions. I foresee the day when physicians will prescribe information. Yes, information. Instead of handing our patients a brochure, which without verbal instruction is not good form, web-savvy doctors will follow up by sending patients an e-mail with informative links back to the doctor's website. If your doctor doesn't have a website with information, ask if the doctor recommends any particular sites where you can read more about your condition or procedure. [*Please see chapter 3 for a more detailed discussion of health/medical websites.*]

- **Patients want to see and understand their conditions.** Most patients and families are fascinated by X-rays, MRIs, CT scans, PET scans, and bone scans. You are entitled to see what your imaging studies look like. By seeing the broken wrist or breast tumor, you can visualize what's going on with you. These pictures really are worth a thousand words when it comes to understanding your illness or condition. Ask the doctor to show you your imaging studies, and also to explain them. Doctors should point out the fractured wrist, the shadow on the mammogram, the blocked coronary artery, the arthritic changes causing knee pain.

- **The doctor does not always know best.** Many patients are too frightened to ask questions, and some still believe that the doctor knows best. We don't. But we try to develop a relationship with our patients so that there is a partnership in protecting your health and attacking a common foe if need be. Patients know when something isn't quite right. We doctors need to listen to what our patients tell us. Many times what we call a "chief complaint" —such as fatigue—

may, in fact, be depression reflecting marital or financial problems.

- **Doctors can make mistakes.** You can guard against being an innocent victim. One woman's X-ray showed a dark shadow on her lung. There was discussion among her doctors about additional diagnostic testing perhaps leading to major surgery. It wasn't until another doctor carefully examined the patient, including a physical inspection of her chest, and discovered that a thick mole on her breast was the cause of the shadow on the X-ray. The physical exam is so crucial in interpreting any imaging tool, such as X-rays or CT scans. I've seen people tentatively diagnosed with cancer when, in fact, the "spots" on the X-rays turned out to be the sticky rectangles of a TENS unit (a small box designed to deliver electrical impulses to people with chronic pain). Make sure the doctor looks at *you,* not just at your X-ray.

- **Doctors know how long you'll be in the hospital, even if they tell you they don't.** Patients always ask me, "How long will I be in the hospital?" Doctors try to avoid answering this one, but they do know in general terms. When you are admitted for a diagnosis, there is always a ballpark figure for the number of days for that diagnosis. I think it's important for you to know how long you might be confined because you have to make arrangements for child care, elder care, work, or feeding the dog. If you can see the end of the tunnel, you can be better prepared. Pin the doctor down by asking, "For someone with my admitting diagnosis, what is the average length of stay in the hospital?" There's always an answer to that question.

- **Doctors don't know the costs of medical care.** You might be given a prescription for an antidepressant the doctor thinks will work for you. Fine. When you are standing at the pharmacy counter and are told the particular brand name of the drug is not covered by your insurance company's formulary (and costs $180), what do you do? Many people have learned that doctors don't have a clue about costs, so before you leave the exam room, discuss generic drug options for the same medication (and you might find your cost is $4 instead of $180). Or, have the pharmacist call the doctor to discuss less costly options. Pharmaceutical reps often give doctors discount coupons for expensive medications; ask your doctor if these are available for necessary medications with no generic option.

I was astounded to learn that my son's surgery on his finger—a procedure we both knew was fairly simple and could be done on an outpatient basis—would cost $14,000. We didn't take courses in medical care finances in medical school. Talk money with the medical practice's office manager. Most patients never do—but they should, especially now.

Understanding Tradition and Culture

A patient is not simply a medical chart or "the lady with colon cancer in room 2307." All patients bring to the bedside their culture, their heritage, their history, and, perhaps, centuries of generational abuse and neglect, and the results of poverty, war, and displacement. Physicians need to understand these issues when treating any patient for any condition. It is especially essential for us to be sensitive to everything about a patient, particularly when we're talking about a life-changing disease.

Mrs. C., for example, was a 73-year-old grandmother from an Asian country who was visiting her family in upstate New York. While there, she developed severe back pain. A biopsy revealed an aggressive cancer which arose from the lung. She had received an appropriate program of radiation therapy at a major medical center and was relatively pain-free. However, because of increasing pain and because of a previous evaluation at the Mayo Clinic, she and her family arrived in Rochester, and I met her in the exam room.

A very careful physical examination demonstrated weakness of the lower limbs, and an MRI of the spine demonstrated an obvious tumor pressing on the spinal cord. It was not possible to provide additional radiation therapy without major damage to the spinal cord. Conferences with gifted and compassionate surgeons led to a grim conclusion: Surgery would not be possible because of the extent of the cancer.

We treated her aggressively with steroid medication to decrease swelling around the tumor, in the hopes of buying time. Chemotherapy was not appropriate because the tumor was resistant to all known forms of therapy.

That's the medical part.

Mrs. C. spoke no English. Likewise, the daughter who accompanied her spoke only an Asian dialect. Fortunately, one of our chief residents was fluent in the patient's language, so let me share with you what unfolded.

We learned that it was not appropriate to mention the word *cancer* because the family was fearful that she would "give up and lose all hope." So we agreed to the family's wishes and used the word *tumor*, which was quite acceptable. Indeed, we do learn from patients.

When dealing with people from all parts of the world—of which we have very little knowledge—it is always appropriate to ask the responsible family member how some of these issues should be handled. The word *cancer* can have devastating implications in some cultures, and so it needs to be appropriately reframed within the context of sharing with the family the potential seriousness of the situation. This is not deceit; this is appropriate compassion and cultural humility, recognizing the ancestral nuances of many patients.

The art and science of treatment

We in Rochester have seen a remarkable increase in individuals from East Africa, especially Somalia. These patients bring to the heartland of Minnesota cultures and traditions and histories that are very different from those of the typical Midwesterner. It is not appropriate in some circumstances for a male physician to extend his hand, and it is also not appropriate for discussions to be directed at the female patient. Decisions of great magnitude typically are filtered through and made by the responsible man of the family, who might be a brother, a father, or a husband.

We need to understand that patients are not always like us. We need to be sensitive to cultural issues and to home in on how these difficult issues should be addressed in different cultures.

As an institution, we've had great experience with members of the Southeast Asian community. Again, issues of health and wellness are treated differently among patients from some of those countries. The physician is viewed as the healer with all knowledge of illness. Therefore, it is bizarre to them when physicians inquire and probe to obtain a medical history from the patient. Their expectation is, "I come to you for help. You have all the answers. So why are you questioning me?"

I received a vivid lesson in this during a trip to Ireland. I had the opportunity to speak in the west coast city of Galway. I was impressed with how the Irish dealt with the diagnosis of advanced cancer. In most circumstances, the elderly patients displayed a sense of peace and acceptance, believed in an afterlife, and quietly accepted the recommendations of their physicians to treat symptoms and to focus on quality of life.

Many patients graciously accepted this news and were prepared to leave the hospital and return home after thanking the caregivers for their guidance and compassion. What a contrast to many American situations in which I see a frantic race to the airport to fly off and seek the elusive medical Holy Grail when, in fact, time might be more profitably spent at home.

The patient we see today may well reflect hundreds or thousands of years of history, culture, oppression, and tradition. We need to recognize that some members of our community may distrust traditional medicine. We need to understand this, and we need to walk with each individual and support the decisions with which he or she is comfortable. No, doctors don't always know best. We learn from our patients every day.

An F in Medical School

You've heard the joke: What do they call the student who graduates last in the class in medical school? The answer is "doctor." But, frankly, we doctors often fail to recognize the needs of our patients. We need to know you. We need to ask questions. And it's reasonable for you to hold us accountable.

We are also not prophets or visionaries. Let us agree to view our interaction as doctor and patient with respectful engagement. We doctors owe that to you, our patients.

How to Be an Empowered Patient

*Only one person truly cares about your health and welfare,
and that's you.*

Americans were shocked by the headline: *Being a patient in the hospital can be hazardous to your health.* A national study in 1999 from the Institute of Medicine reported that approximately 98,000 patients die each year as a result of medical mistakes made in hospitals. A report as recently as 2013 said 70,000 people die in hospitals. (Many of these deaths are from the infection known as sepsis.) But a report in the *Journal of Patient Safety* put the number well over 400,000, making medical errors the third leading cause of death, behind heart disease and cancer.

Obviously, these numbers generate much concern. The types of errors noted were misread lab reports, blood mismatched during transfusions, wrong prescriptions given to the wrong person or in the wrong dose, and wrong-site surgery, which is removing the left leg or left kidney, for example, when it was the right leg or right kidney (or similarly paired body organ) that was diseased.

Hospitals Can Be Dangerous Places

Infections acquired in hospitals can be deadly. The CDC says half of these infections can be prevented by proper hand washing. Whose job is it to police the care provider in hand washing? The patient's? But doctors and nurses wear gloves, you say. Yes, gloves have become ever-present, yet gloves are designed to protect the wearer, not you. Gloves can surely spread germs if they become contaminated, just like a bare hand. Think about it.

Regardless of the type of error—wrong-site surgery or insufficient hand washing—medical error is a serious problem in hospitals today. But just what has caused this problem? There are as many answers as there are experts in this area, but let me take a stab at it. Keep in mind I'm trying to explain some reasons behind this problem, knowing that there is no excuse for medical error.

The body of medical information in scientific research journals is doubling approximately every 24 to 36 months. New drugs are launched into the marketplace daily. Therefore, it is impossible for any single medical professional to keep up to date with all the latest developments. This is especially important when patients receive many kinds of medications, particularly because some of these may interact with one another in dangerous ways.

Patients need to be proactive about learning and clearly understanding the dosages, frequencies, and reasons for the medications that they are taking. But patients and families cannot be expected to understand the complex interactions among a variety of medications. This is why physicians, pharmacists, and nurses work closely to monitor any bad side effects or interactions which may occur when medications react to one another inside the body.

Likewise, as discussed earlier, a clear doctor-patient dialogue should occur about what medications are being prescribed and taken. Rather than add another medication to an already long list, we physicians need to be challenged to reduce medications to the absolute minimum.

At the same time that medical care is advancing, medical devices are increasing in their complexity. Biopsies are now being performed on parts of the body that were never accessible in the past. Through the techniques of ultrasound-guided biopsies and CT-scan-guided biopsies, tiny pieces of tissue can be extracted from organs, such as the pancreas, and also from lymph nodes buried deep in the abdominal or pelvic cavities. In the past, some patients required a major abdominal operation to secure this type of tissue.

These procedures can now be performed much more safely. Various types of tubes can be placed into intestinal cavities, and these may pose risks for infection. Intravenous dye tests are now routinely used; whereas, formerly, these had been part of medical diagnoses only infrequently. But every invasive test, from the taking of blood to a major operation, poses risks for the patient. Know and understand your risks.

We are in the midst of a national nursing shortage too. Some nurses are working back-to-back shifts, and a 12-hour shift is not at all uncommon. We need to acknowledge that a fatigue factor exists.

Obviously, the patient and the family cannot be expected to make an impact on the national shortage of nurses. However, patients and families can be vigilant and participate with the nursing staff in major decisions. You may (and should) ask the nurse taking care of you why a medication is being given. It is your right to know why a certain test is sensible. If the answers to these questions simply don't feel right or if you have a level of discomfort, it would be prudent to ask for reassurance or clarification from another member of the nursing team.

Another option: If you (or a family member) feel a problem has emerged that will require evaluation in the hospital or in the emergency room, it makes good sense to try to make the visit as early as possible in the day. Realistically, this may not always be feasible, because illnesses and accidents don't follow the clock. But if you have the option, it is probably far better to seek medical guidance during the light of day than to walk into the emergency room at 3:00 a.m.

We're not number 1

It is fairly common knowledge that, despite our medical advances in medications and technology, as a country, we are not doing well in health care. According to a study in *JAMA,* we as a country have ranked last or near the bottom in areas of infant mortality, years of potential life lost, and life expectancy for men.

What is especially dreadful is that iatrogenic injuries are the third leading cause of death in the United States, after heart disease and cancer. The term *iatrogenic* means "caused by medical intervention."

In other words, the patient was harmed because of the treatment. It's not a fun discussion in physician groups.

Now how can this be? As a practicing physician with daily responsibilities for patients in the hospital as well as in the clinic, I will map out what typically may occur. When you're in the hospital (and I have been a patient myself, so I know), a platoon of providers interacts with you, the patient. People from the lab come and take blood; nurses and others take your temperature and blood pressure more often than you'd like. Your doctor and maybe residents or medical students examine you. Staff members will transport you in wheelchairs or beds. Assistants may help you to the bathroom. Others hand you medications.

Each of these individuals is a vector for potential infection. We each know about the importance of appropriate hand washing, but in the midst of the many pressures of working in a busy hospital, sometimes this is not always done.

As a patient, you have rights, and one of those rights is to ask everyone—*everyone*—who touches you to wash his or her hands first, and to do so in front of you.

Patients Have Rights, Too

Your doctor may be in charge of your care when you're in the hospital, but you're still in charge of you. If you're in the hospital as a patient, you *do* have control over what happens to you, even though you may think you're at the mercy of anyone who pokes and prods you. Patients hate to be awakened at 4:00 a.m. for a blood pressure reading. They really don't like to be stuck for blood five times a day. Most patients put up with this because they think they don't have control over it.

Well, you do have control. You do have rights. Every hospital has a patient's bill of rights. If you aren't given a copy when you come in, ask for one. Negotiate with the nursing staff. Tell them you do not want to be awakened if you are asleep—at any time of day. The lead nurse is your best advocate. Find out who this person is, and make sure you both agree that if blood has to be drawn for different doctors, the lab draws it all at once. Bring a family member or friend to be your advocate because you're not on top of your game. Hey, you're in the hospital.

Hospitals have visiting hours, but that's to prevent anyone and everyone from traipsing into your room and invading your privacy at any hour of the day or night. Nothing prevents you from having a close friend or family member sitting by your bedside monitoring your activities anytime, helping you with the little things like getting water or changing the TV channel, as long as this person doesn't get in the way of your care. Especially if you're just coming out of anesthesia or are quite weak and unable to truly communicate your needs, I recommend that you have your advocate at your side.

It's sensible to be appropriately inquisitive and proactive and to participate with the health care providers. Ask your targeted questions, such as the ones listed here and elsewhere in this book. During times of high stress and anxiety, it's impossible for any of us to remember what we wanted to ask and then to remember the doctor's answer. That's why I always recommend that an advocate or a family member or a confidante accompany the patient and act on that patient's behalf with the patient's permission.

You will be asked to sign an informed consent sheet for many procedures. You will receive a copy of this form to remind you of the discussions and what you can anticipate about the treatment duration, the possible side effects, and whom to contact if a complication occurs. Don't sign until all your questions are answered.

Patients always have questions about their upcoming procedures or surgeries. They want to know when their stitches will be taken out or when they can return to work. We are asked all kinds of questions, and a doctor or other health care practitioner should be prepared to answer any and all questions patiently. An effortless way out for some health care providers is to give you easy-to-understand handouts and pamphlets addressing the specifics of many procedures—from appendectomy to vasectomy. Many medical offices have these types of patient-education tools available in print format and even on DVD.

But for a doctor or other health care provider to simply hand you a brochure and not be available to answer your questions is not ideal. The informed patient is better positioned to get the maximum benefit from care. It is fair for you to ask for a copy of the hospital discharge summary.

Speak Up

Again, the Institute of Medicine has clearly documented that thousands of patients die each year from preventable and avoidable medical mistakes. Programs are now being crafted to monitor this situation, but what can *you* do in the meantime?

- Ask questions. Never assume that everyone taking part in your care knows all the details about you and your medical history, including any allergies or bad reactions, especially to medications.
- Ask about the dosages of each medication, how often it is to be given, and the anticipated duration of treatment, at the time each one is prescribed.
- Understand your treatment. For example, some types of chemotherapy are administered over six to eight hours on an outpatient basis. If one of your treatments is completed in two hours rather than six hours, you need to inquire as to why this change in the schedule has occurred.
- If you're in the hospital and a health care practitioner hands you a pill, don't take it until that person checks your ID bracelet. Imagine what would happen if the person in the bed next to you has the same or similar name. Ask questions: What is this pill? What is this for? If your regular blood pressure pills are yellow and the nurse brings you a blue pill, ask before you swallow. If the technician is hanging a new IV bag with medication or blood, is your name on that bag? Check first.
- Having surgery? Surgeons now are signing their name on the site of your anticipated incision before you are put under anesthesia. If the biopsy is on your left breast, for example, you might even have the nurse write "NO" on surgical tape and place it across your right breast.
- If the doctor writes you a prescription and you can't read it, don't presume that the pharmacist can. Ask the name of

the medication, what it is for, and how often you are to take it. Confirm all these details with the pharmacist when you have the prescription filled. And make sure the prescription you are given is for you. Is your name on the bottle? If this is a refill, do the pills look the same as last time?

- From a practical standpoint, understanding what you can expect when entering the hospital as a patient is important. That way, you may know if something isn't quite right. Ask questions like these: *Do I have to be fasting for certain tests? What will happen to me before surgery and after surgery? Do you expect that I will be receiving blood or antibiotics following surgery or while in the hospital? If so, how much blood will I be receiving? Over what time will it be given? What is the name of the antibiotic, and what is the dose and frequency?* And have someone with you, if possible, at all times.

Don't (Always) Believe the Headlines

The Internet has, of course, changed everything related to receiving and disseminating information. More information than you ever thought possible is at your command by keystroke or mouse click. As I've mentioned already, trust only sites maintained by credible organizations, and use the information you find to guide, not replace, your discussions with your health care providers,

Sometimes your morning newspaper or evening TV news may be your source for medical information, and therein may lie a problem.

The cure for cancer is on *The Today Show*. At least that's what you thought you heard. Advances in medical treatment make headline news every day. Local TV anchors do what are called "cut-ins" to tease you to stay tuned for your local news. They'll mention the "new cure for *[insert disease name here]* " or the "breakthrough treatment that's saving lives." You stay tuned, you listen, and you eventually (maybe) hear that the so-called breakthrough took place in a laboratory rat, and the technology is still years from being tried on humans, if it ever gets that far.

Let's separate hope from hype.

The gap between what's going on in the laboratory and actual clinical practice is wide. Additionally, the media often are quick to latch onto what they think are scientific truths, when, in fact, the science behind "a cure" is evolving slowly and taking its academic and clinical time. No one told us in medical school that our patients would challenge us about something they heard on cable news or read online.

Medical news can be confusing. By the time a clinical study gets into your local newspaper, the information has gone through so many filters, you can't be sure you're getting the whole story. The bottom line for you is the answer to this question: *What does this information mean to me?*

Journalists would be wise to avoid charged words, such as *breakthrough* and *medical miracle*, although such overblown descriptions are enticing and boost ratings and readership. Words like that should rarely be used in mainstream medical news coverage. Medicine is advancing, but in slow, steady increments. The *cure* for cancer or diabetes or multiple sclerosis is not going to pop into tomorrow's headlines.

The forerunner to any cure is happening today in laboratories and in clinics through clinical trials. Preliminary results are written and then circulated to experts in the field. If judged credible, the studies are reported in peer-reviewed medical journals. This process takes months, even years, and none of us involved in medical research would ever characterize our work as a "medical miracle." We have many failures you never read about in the headlines.

The only place to read headlines about a cure for cancer or the common cold is in a supermarket tabloid. And while some Internet chat rooms or forums may be abuzz with talk of wiping out the West Nile Virus or Ebola, it's just not going to happen quickly.

The problem comes when journalists misinterpret preliminary findings and then make the leap from the laboratory to mainstream medical practice, raising false hopes. Medical breakthroughs are not leaps at all, but slow deliberate steps.

Can You Believe
What You Read in the Headlines?

I suggest you follow these guidelines in evaluating the headlines in the news media and then judge for yourself:

Was the study performed by responsible, credentialed investigators at a major center?

Now don't misunderstand me. Sometimes the obscure researcher in a relatively unheard of institution may find a key piece of the puzzle. However, that is unusual. So if you do not recognize the name of the institution, university, or medical center, or if you do not recognize the credentials of the researcher, you need to be cautious.

Was the vaccine or drug analyzed in a randomized clinical trial?

In other words, were some patients given a new drug and others given standard treatment in order to sort out whether or not the vaccine/drug really works or is better than standard treatment? Without a test group and a group to compare, it's hard to say something "works."

How many patients received the treatment?

In order to determine the benefit from a treatment (such as surgery or a drug), it is highly likely that hundreds of patients are needed in a clinical trial. If the number is limited to a dozen or so people with the same disease or condition, you need to be suspicious of the results. Were humans used at all, or was this a research study conducted with laboratory animals?

Who is the sponsor?

If the press release or the news commentary is exclusively sponsored by a drug company, you need to carefully interpret the data. Our colleagues in the pharmaceutical industry are in partnership with medical practitioners. Few institutions, such as medical centers or universities, have the resources to conduct research without financial support. We need to cooperate and collaborate with input from the pharmaceutical industry. However, we also need to recognize that we live in the real world, and sometimes economic motives may artificially inflate the benefit from the treatment.

How was the trial conducted?

In other words, every patient receiving the treatment needs to be accounted for. Let's suppose the press story indicated that the benefit occurred in 50 percent of patients who took a flu vaccine. Something happened with the others, and was that significant?

The pace of medical research can be maddeningly slow, and it is not likely that a researcher laboring in some underground bunker will come forward with the home-run therapy for diseases X, Y, or Z. Science simply does not work that way.

From a cancer perspective, let's focus on the interferon story.

Decades ago, this medication appeared on the cover of *Time* magazine. Interferon was heralded as the answer for cancer, as well as a whole host of other disorders, such as multiple sclerosis and hepatitis. Study after study carefully addressed the value of this agent, and yet, at the present time, the high hopes for this medication have been disappointing. We now know that interferon can be a toxic medication, and its value applies only to a very small number of patients with some highly unusual diseases. The lesson: We need to be cautious, we need to be somewhat cynical, and we need to be suspicious when a home-run therapy is touted in the news.

Let's shift gears for a moment and look at coronary artery disease, the number 1 killer in America. For decades, medical dogma has clearly focused on the role of cholesterol as a major factor in blocking the arteries. There is rock-solid scientific evidence that cholesterol is a major factor in causing heart attacks. But hold on, new blood studies are focusing on inflammation as a factor in heart disease and a substance in the blood called C-reactive protein, which may point toward individuals at high risk for a heart attack even if they have normal cholesterol levels. Science is always questioning itself; that's the nature of inquiry.

Consider ulcers. For centuries we believed that ulcers were related to stress and undoubtedly were related to a weakening in the wall of the stomach that allowed acid to erode a hole in the stomach. "Don't get stressed or you'll get an ulcer" was the reasoning. We now know that ulcers are caused by infectious germs—not stress—and antibiotics are part of mainstream therapy for ulcer disease. Stress? I'm not sure where we go with that now. Stress can be hazardous to your health, of course. For ulcers, however, you'll probably have to blame them on something other than your boss or your family!

So how can we separate hype from actual hope?

Let me take you behind some of the real headlines from mainstream newspapers and magazines (not supermarket tabloids), so next time you read or hear about a so-called cure or other breakthrough, you can judge for yourself.

This story is about chicken soup and the common cold. There's something about chicken soup that just makes you feel better when you're sneezing and sniffling through a winter cold. Is it the loving care Mom provides along with the soup? Could it be the steamy aroma and nutrient-rich broth? Could it be something else?

Scientists at the University of Nebraska Medical Center studied "Grandma's soup" prepared by the lead researcher's wife from a family recipe—in the laboratory under carefully controlled conditions.

Although common colds are not completely understood, it is believed that the inflammation caused when the body defends itself against infection could be blocked by the chicken soup. And that is indeed what Stephen Rennard, M.D., and his colleagues found—*in test tubes*.

If soup can reduce inflammation in test tubes, which researchers measured in the lab, it *might* reduce the symptoms of a cold in humans. Theory. Speculation. Something to study further.

The results were published a decade ago by the American College of Chest Physicians in the journal *Chest,* and these support what some may consider food-as-medicine theory. And the headlines proclaimed, of course, that chicken soup cures the common cold. That's not what the scientists found; that's what overly enthusiastic news reporters mistakenly interpreted. Much of the resultant media frenzy didn't even mention that the findings were restricted to cold germs in test tubes.

The university press relations people had great fun in an out-of-control situation, and as part of their damage control, they put Grandma's soup recipe on the university's website. In this case, no damage was done, and people with colds that winter were probably making plenty of chicken soup.

I have a few other favorites to tell you about:

- *The Los Angeles Times* reported on a promising cancer drug over a decade ago. When I first wrote this book in 2003, I said this: **Drug aims to inhibit cancer by altering cell environment.** This drug is called Velcade (bortezomib), and its potential use is for patients with multiple myeloma, a type of bone marrow cancer. The initial studies appeared promising, but this is generally the case because patients participating in early clinical trials like this one usually are carefully selected. This particular medication is of great interest because it blocks a series of enzymes that are involved with cell division. In early laboratory studies, this medication induced cell death. However, we must await a long-term study involving hundreds of patients before the verdict is finally in. And now, 10 years later, the verdict is in and the news is good. The point is that it took 10 years at least.

- Data from the National Cancer Institute were presented with this headline: **Shark cancers cast more doubt on cartilage pills.** Sharks are supposed to have super immune systems and apparently do not get cancer, so whatever sharks have should be used to treat cancers in humans. Or so the theory went. In this study, government scientists were attempting to disprove the value of shark cartilage as a cancer cure. This study confirms clinical studies at Mayo Clinic and other organizations, all of which show that shark cartilage offers no value, other than to fuel the false hopes of desperate patients. Our results were negative. Shark cartilage has no effect, and, apparently, sharks *do* get cancer. Even with major medical centers disproving its value, shark cartilage is still big business. You can do a global Internet search and find hundreds of websites that will sell you capsules and powders of shark cartilage, with each site claiming the product cures cancer. Without a randomized, controlled trial, so-called cures are pure speculation. Until these hucksters show you the science, please don't show them your money.

Are there really advances? Yes, of course. Advances in the treatment of cancer are agonizingly slow, have many false stops and starts, and lead even the most conscientious scientist down multiple dead ends. However, with persistence, tenacity, and a little good luck, some striking findings are now being developed and reported in the headlines.

About 40 years ago, patients with chronic myeloid leukemia were discovered to have an unusual chromosome entitled the Philadelphia chromosome. A specific enzyme is detected in almost all cases of chronic myeloid leukemia, and also in a smaller proportion of patients with acute lymphoblastic leukemia. Several years ago, scientists published a fascinating study on the role of a chemical initially named ST1571, now called Gleevec. This medication specifically blocked or deactivated an enzyme called tyrosine kinase, which was present in the patients with these two forms of leukemia. The findings were striking in that more than half of these patients with each form of leukemia had remarkable benefits, and the side effects were quite manageable and tolerable. These findings suggested that there could be "targeted therapy" or "smart treatments."

These findings have now been extended to patients with other cancers, most notably an unusual form called gastrointestinal stromal tumors. Again, the results have been striking and the side effects relatively modest. In other words, in this case there is a "heat-seeking missile" that goes directly to the cancer cells, rather than a nonspecific treatment such as chemotherapy, which attacks all rapidly dividing cells, both malignant and nonmalignant, and causes a whole host of side effects (nausea, vomiting, risks of bleeding, and infection).

Believe me, researchers are hunched over their microscopes conducting intense studies to determine the value of this type of medication in a variety of other cancers.

The lesson is that the tireless efforts of scientists in laboratories throughout the country, at some point in time, have the potential of providing the key to unlock the secrets of cancer and other diseases. We need to be realistic. It is not likely that one medication and the interruption of one enzyme will apply to all cancers, but the Gleevec story truly is a success story (but not an overnight success story) in which we can all take hope from the headlines.

My Prevention Rx

Medicine is changing at a blistering pace. No one practitioner can know all there is to know on any one subject. But you can know everything you need to know about you. Whether you're a patient in the doctor's office or a patient in a hospital, getting a new prescription, or having a regular checkup, it's critical for you to be your own best watchdog and advocate. As an informed patient, you and your family can better partner with your health care providers to get the best results as you journey down whatever path is in store for you—whether because of your medical history, sudden illness or injury, or any other circumstance.

When your search for medical knowledge takes you to mainstream media, understand the minefields and be skeptical about the headlines. Articles published in peer-reviewed medical journals are just that—communication among members of the scientific world who are exchanging ideas and findings. Sometimes this information becomes headline news when, in reality, it's not ready for prime time. The Internet allows even more users (not just medical personnel) to access medical information and journals that they never would have read in the past.

Opening this medical world is helpful if used and interpreted in context, but when laboratory findings among 14 volunteers in Finland become headline news in Cedar Rapids, Iowa, the problems crop up in doctors' offices across the country. When science and the media give mixed signals, our patients get their hopes up, and we doctors are left to explain the cold, harsh reality.

PART TWO

Good Health by Choice,
Not Chance

6

What Should I Get Screened For?

Knowledge changes behavior.
Knowledge empowers us.
Knowledge can save our lives.

This is the I-hate-going-to-the-doctor-when-nothing-is-wrong chapter. I always cringe at the analogy many writers make comparing the human body to a car. You don't ignore the warning lights on the dashboard or the oil drips on the garage floor. So why ignore your body's aches, pains, spots, and dots?

Some months ago, on a Sunday morning, a prominent professional called me with this opening statement: "Sally has breast cancer, in the liver, and we were told she has about four months to live. We are overwhelmed and need help. My God, what do we do, how did this happen?" Not science fiction, real life. Tragically, this could have been prevented. How? With a yearly mammogram and a professional physical examination of the breast.

True scenario number two. My stepfather called me late one bitterly cold winter night. He was hoarse, weak, and frightened, had blood in his phlegm, and was short of breath. He had been a heavy smoker for 40 years. He was dead within nine weeks of that call.

What happened to him? Same story. Studies now show that long-term smokers have a better survival rate from lung cancer if they get screening CT scans before the cancer gets so advanced that cure is not possible.

Almost all of us buckle up in the car—or know we should. Many of us use helmets when biking—or know we should. And almost all of us seek shelter inside during a lightning storm. Why? Because we know that it makes good sense to be safe. Knowledge changes behavior. Knowledge empowers us.

Let me get personal for a moment. I know, on a daily basis, the challenge of treating advanced cancer of the colon and rectum. I know that this disease is curable, preventable, and beatable if, and only if, detected early. So I discussed having a colonoscopy with my doctor. We agreed that when I reached age 50, a screening of the entire colon would be sensible. My Easter dinner that year was a gallon of fluids to clean out my colon for the test the next day. The screening was not a big deal, and all was well. But I had positioned myself to detect a disease that could be fatal.

We all need to reduce our risks—whether by wearing a helmet or getting our colons checked—so we can go the distance. We can arm ourselves with knowledge and then take action. At the track we back the horse with a proven track record to handle the slop (muddy surface) or to go the distance. Same philosophy with our health, except we do *not* get a second chance with our health.

Give Your Doctor a Checkup First

I talk with my doctor about what I should do. Sure, I'm a doctor, but we all need a partner in our own health. This partnership is not only important, it's critical. We need to be active participants, not passive consumers. We are not buying a car. We are "buying" (selecting and paying the fee of) the person we will entrust to protect our health and life. That's why I suggest you check out your doctor before you get a checkup.

After all, you price TV sets before you buy. You shop around for automobiles. You try on clothes. Why not "try on" a new doctor to see if the chemistry is right? In this chapter, you'll learn the ins and outs of doctor shopping—what credentials to look for, how to check on the doctor's reputation, and whom to believe—even if your choices are limited by your insurance network. Even with emerging changes in health care reform, we may not have unlimited access to the provider of our choice.

You may seek a new doctor for a number of reasons: your doctor moves or retires, you move and want a medical office closer to where you live, or you change health plans and might have to choose a doctor from a selected list. You might just be unhappy with your current doctor. And the list goes on.

Sometimes you will require a doctor with a particular specialty, such as when you get pregnant and need an obstetrician, and then have a child and need a pediatrician. Other times, you just want another opinion, or are dissatisfied and want better care. Whatever your reason for seeking a new doctor, you'll want to choose a physician you trust and with whom you are comfortable.

The best time to choose a doctor is when you *don't* need one. Just like you don't want to be looking through the yellow pages for a lawyer if you're arrested, you don't want to be searching for a doctor when you have a medical emergency. Check out the doctor first to make sure he or she is licensed in your state, has the training you require, and has board certification. You can even find out where the doctor had medical training and in what specialties. All this information is online.

Here's where to start:

- Ask your family, friends, and coworkers if they would recommend their doctors—and why they would or wouldn't. These are often reliable sources.
- Community hospitals and large medical centers often have "Find-a-Doctor" phone referral centers. These are reasonable places to begin the journey of finding a health care provider. Once you and your family have the names of physicians or providers, it certainly would be appropriate to check their credentials.
- Your health plan, whether it's a managed network or some other provider plan, may publish (in print or online) a directory of providers in the plan. This is another list to narrow your search online. The doctor's or clinic's own website should contain physician and staff bios.
- Some states have websites where you can access any medical professionals who might have disciplinary action pending.

Simply because a doctor is being sued does not mean that the physician is not qualified, compassionate, and thorough.

- Conduct a national search through the site of the American Medical Association at *ama-assn.org*. You can search by physician name or medical specialty. To locate a doctor near you, enter your ZIP code. You'll find out where the doctor trained, his or her specialties, and whether he or she is board certified.

- Look for a board-certified doctor. Go to the American Board of Medical Specialties at *abms.org*. Click "Who's Certified," and follow the form. You may also simply ask the doctor or the office staff, or look at the framed certificates on the walls at your current doctor's office. Board certification indicates a basic level of training and expertise.

What board certification means

The kind of specialized training a doctor has had in treating your condition does matter. Board certification is a credential or an acknowledgment of expertise that the doctor has taken and passed a test on a fundamental body of knowledge. Always look for "board certification" in the specialty related to your condition when you are seeking a well-trained physician. This is a prerequisite.

If a doctor is a member of a medical specialty society and has board certification, the doctor may have additional letters following his or her name (an example would be John Doe, M.D., F.A.C.S., meaning Dr. Doe is a Fellow of the American College of Surgeons). Because I am board certified in hospice and palliative medicine and am a fellow in that organization, I can use F.A.A.H.P.M. after my M.D. This means that I am a Fellow in the American Academy of Hospice and Palliative Medicine. Look for similar designations (these really are rigorous accomplishments that many docs don't have). Palliative, by the way, means relieving and preventing suffering of patients who may or may not be in hospice or end-of-life care.

This additional certification assures you that the doctor has demonstrated expertise in a specialty area. Not every doctor has board certification. A doctor who does not have board certification may not have taken the "boards"—the certification test. Or may have taken the exam and failed.

Credentials—a confusing alphabet soup

Now, how to make some sense of the bewildering alphabet soup of credentials? Most of us recognize the initials for the M.D. (doctor of medicine) or D.O. (doctor of osteopathy), as well as the Ph.D. (doctor of philosophy) and R.N. (registered nurse). The P.A. is a physician assistant, and the N.P. is a nurse-practitioner. Both are highly qualified to work under the guidance of your doctor. You may see a C.N.M. (certified nurse midwife) or F.N.P (family nurse-practitioner). For counseling issues, you may work with an M.S.W. (master of social work) or Psy.D. (doctor of psychology). But a host of other professionals with credentials may play a role in the management of your health.

The physical therapist (P.T.) and the doctor of chiropractic (D.C.) are two kinds of professionals who may indeed provide care for you. If you are not familiar with a caregiver's credentials and area of expertise, it might be appropriate to ask for his or her professional credentials and training. If the practitioner is part of your managed care network, you can almost be assured that he or she has been checked out.

Be warned. Some so-called professionals with questionable credentials should not be on your medical management team.

How can you tell the difference?

Anyone worth working with will readily comply if you ask about certification. If the person you are consulting has no state or national licensure board that has approved him or her to practice, you need to be concerned. The beauty of the Internet is that it allows you to go to the organization's website and check out the credibility online. If the "credential" is just a course completed during a weekend at a Holiday Inn Express, beware.

If the practitioner with the unusual credentials expects a large "up front" cash advance, or if the person is practicing in a foreign country, you need to be realistic and have legitimate amounts of suspicion. Framed diplomas or fancy letters after someone's name doesn't give them a free pass to practice on you or on your family.

Making the final choice

Your final decision in choosing among doctors who are equally trained may come down to personality and practice style. Choose a doctor who communicates well with you. Make an appointment just to meet a potential new doctor.

Ask (and get satisfactory answers to) these questions before you schedule your appointment:

- Are the office hours and location convenient? Is parking available nearby?
- Who covers for the doctor when he or she is off, or after hours?
- Is the office and nursing staff courteous? How hard is it to get an appointment when needed or if urgent?
- Will the doctor be a partner with you in your care? Are you listened to? Do you feel validated and acknowledged or dismissed and ignored? These are big issues.
- What about insurance coverage? Who files the insurance forms?

If you feel comfortable with the doctor after checking out the credentials and training, and after meeting the doctor—with your clothes on—trust your instincts. You've probably found the right partner.

The Doctor Doesn't Always Know Best— You Do

Nationwide polls point to cancer as the number 1 health concern. Yet despite our concern for this dreaded disease (and others), we often ignore the risk factors in our lives, choose not to follow cancer-prevention diets and lifestyles, think cancer may be inevitable if we have a strong family history of the disease, or don't know how often to be screened for cancer. All these points are clearly made in health polls.

Yet the fact remains that heart disease—not cancer—will kill more of us than any other disease. Nonetheless, women fear breast and ovarian cancers and skin cancer far out of proportion to their actual risk of dying of these types of cancer. Men are most concerned about prostate and lung cancers. Yet neither men nor women are as concerned about cancers of the colon and rectum (the third most deadly for both genders) as they should be.

What is the single most important determinant of whether you will develop cancer? If you said family history, you are wrong. It's your age and, to some extent, your lifestyle and life choices. As you age, your risk increases.

You can't control your age, but you can control another factor that plays a very large part in the development of cancer. Two-thirds of cancer deaths are related to one issue. Would you like to guess? It's lifestyle, especially diet—two practices you can control. Which explains why age and lifestyle should be considered when you discuss your medical history with your doctor. You can reduce your risk with early detection and screening, but how often you need certain tests is still not commonly known.

The American Cancer Society recommends a cancer-related checkup every three years for men and women between 20 and 39, and every year once you hit 40. Chances are you have never had a specific cancer-related checkup. To see the various tests you may need and at what ages, go to the website of the American Cancer Society for detailed checklists (*cancer.org,* search "Cancer Screening Guidelines").

General health screenings are also outlined in various places online (one popular place is *MerckEngage.com* [click "Healthy Conversations/Health Screenings"]), so I won't reprint them here, but I will discuss some of the tests and why they are important—and what their limitations are.

Certainly knowing what to do and doing the right things are two different issues, as we discussed earlier in relation to behavior change. Your health plan is now required in almost all circumstances to cover routine screening exams. So the chances are you are now more likely to get these tests.

At one time in medical history, on a fairly regular basis, many patients underwent a comprehensive screening assessment, which often included dangerous, expensive, and inconvenient interventions. I can vividly recall as a young medical student at the University of Michigan caring for executives who were hospitalized for up to five days for stomach X-rays, colon X-rays, and a battery of other studies that certainly could have been done on an outpatient basis. I am not being critical. This was the method of medical practice at that time in history.

Today, however, the annual physical exam has been reconsidered. A careful, targeted, and focused history, together with a physical exam, generally provide the cornerstone of an assessment. Routine blood studies assessing anemia, liver functions, thyroid functions, sugar levels, and levels of cholesterol and triglycerides are reasonable, based on your age, risk factors, and gender.

Appropriate screening studies, such as the mammogram and the colonoscopy, are reasonable. In general today, the "annual physical exam" is much more limited, targeted, and much more focused on your needs rather than on a haphazard "shotgun approach" subjecting you to every new technology.

Early Detection: A Mantra to Follow

A dogma of medicine, which is clearly supported by the literature and by statistics, is that the earlier a condition is detected, the better the probability of a cure and a more positive outcome. Let's suppose an individual has vague chest heaviness or tightness with exertion. This is called angina pectoris (chest pain). If this condition is recognized early, it is conceivable that the patient might have a variety of cardiac assessments clearly defining the problem, and this might be corrected by a bypass procedure or by having a stent inserted into the partially blocked artery leading to the heart. Either procedure can be lifesaving.

In other words, early detection of the problem can result in a resolution of the problem, with continuation of a relatively normal life for the individual.

Now let's look at diabetes. Suppose at the time of an annual physical examination an individual has an elevated blood sugar level. By finding this condition early with a simple blood test, this person can make lifestyle changes through diet and exercise, which can be introduced so that the condition can be controlled, and the patient may very well live a relatively normal life. The hemoglobin A1C is another blood test to assess diabetes.

Consider the situation of a potentially blocked carotid artery. This is an artery in the neck that feeds blood from the heart into the brain. If this artery becomes significantly blocked, the patient may have a stroke resulting in significant disabilities, such as paralysis, blindness, or even death. If this abnormality is detected early enough during a physical exam—as the doctor listens to blood flow in neck arteries and assesses the pulse in the neck—we can perform surgical and medical interventions to correct the problem so that the patient's life can be not only saved, but enhanced.

My take-home message: Early detection for any condition, including cancer, results (in most cases) in a more favorable outcome than if the condition is not found at an earlier stage.

There is no question. We are having a great deal of success in the war against cancer and other dreaded diseases. Today, people are living longer than at any time in history. The successes and the breakthroughs in labs and through clinical trials, however, apply to a very small proportion of cancers. For example, patients with cancers arising from the testicle, which have widely spread, are now curable with chemotherapy, as are some types of lung cancers, especially the small-cell type. Likewise the treatment of some kinds of colon cancer has achieved remarkable success in some patients. Childhood cancers, which were uniformly fatal just a few years ago, are now consistently curable.

Yet for some patients with advanced cancers arising from other areas—gastrointestinal tract, brain, kidney, bladder, lung—the survival rate is not much different now than it was 10 or 15 years ago. In essence, there have been islands of striking success for some patients. For example, select patients with certain lung cancers with a favorable genetic profile may do well, and some patients with a strain of malignant melanoma with a certain genetic marker have excellent short-term success. But when we step back to the 30,000-foot view and survey the landscape of most patients with far-advanced cancer, the progress has been sluggish.

We now have FDA-approved "targeted" therapies for some types of kidney cancer and some types of other advanced cancer, but for most patients the benefits are limited. And these treatments apply to a very small minority of all cancer patients.

This underscores the overarching importance of lifestyle issues and early detection to enhance our ability to cure cancers. Half of all cancers are caused by lifestyle choices. A sedentary lifestyle, a high-fat diet, inappropriate exposure to the sun, obesity, and, obviously, tobacco and alcohol account for about half of cancers. Therefore, if you become empowered, proactive, and assertive, you can shift the odds from the house to your favor by following some commonsense rules of restricting solid fats, being physically active, using sunscreen, not smoking, and restricting alcohol to a minimum.

Now what about early detection and screening? Screening is testing to detect a disease. Detection, therefore, is what happens during or as a result of screening, which may then prevent you from developing a life-threatening illness—all by nabbing it in its early and highly curable stages.

Catching the Number 1 Killer (P.S.: It's Not Cancer)

This bears repeating: Heart disease and stroke are the nation's number 1 killers. So it's no wonder the American Heart Association recommends regular blood pressure checks at least every 2 years, starting at age 20. But being overweight and obese are also clear risk factors for heart disease. Body mass index (BMI) and waist-to-hip comparisons are also measures to assess obesity, but it seems to me that we can do that by looking in the mirror. Keeping your weight in check can be difficult as age seems to creep up on us around our middles. But reasonable and controlled weight gain into middle age can be done.

Measuring weight is routine in any doctor's visit. And so is taking your blood pressure. You can also slide into one of those blood pressure stations next time you're in a drugstore. Many people keep a card in their wallets or purses so that they can write down the date and their blood pressure numbers. I recommend it. It's relatively easy to measure and track your own numbers in these areas.

Cholesterol measurement, including the full lipid profile that includes all types of cholesterol (HDL, LDL, and triglycerides), is another detection tool the American Heart Association recommends every 5 years, starting at age 20. This involves drawing a small sample of blood. You don't have to wait for a doctor's appointment to get these numbers. If you attend a health fair at work or in the community, you can also keep track of these numbers yourself. Certainly if these measures are high, you'll want to discuss them with your doctor right away. Diet and exercise can make a dramatic difference for you.

With a family history of heart disease, however, you'll want to track these measures much more frequently and partner with your doctor in monitoring your risks.

For the cancer doctor, the "fatal four" are cancers of the lung, breast, colon, and prostate. These killers account for more than half of all cancer deaths in the United States. The madness about these cancers is that, in large part, they are preventable, avoidable, and curable if detected at an early stage. Again, this bears repeating.

As I've already mentioned, cancer is the disease the public fears most, which is why screening for cancer is so vital. I'm not downplaying the importance of uncovering a developing glaucoma or high blood sugar, but with cancer, the stakes are high, even life-threatening. So let's cover cancer detection now, and then move toward other conditions that benefit from early detection and treatment.

Which Tests to Have When, and What the Results Mean

Although your doctor should have a record of the tests performed by that medical office, and all those results should be in your medical chart, I advise you to be the keeper of a copy of this information. [*Please see chapter 3 for a more detailed explanation of why you need to maintain your medical records and how to do so.*]

Fecal occult blood test

Cancer of the colon is a major killer in this country. Long-term dietary and population studies strongly hint that diets high in fat and red meat have something to do with the frequency of this disease. Some interesting studies have also indicated that physically active people may decrease their risk of colon cancer. Now why should this be?

It may be related to less contact time between the food we eat and the lining of the colon. Undoubtedly, there are cancer-causing chemicals in what we eat, and by rapidly transporting these materials through the colon, there is a lower frequency of the genetic mutation that may result in cancer.

At one time, the fecal occult blood test was viewed as the gold standard for the evaluation of cancers of the colon and rectum. The theory went something like this: Cancers would typically bleed, and that blood could be detected by smearing a stool specimen on a small piece of cardboard about the size of a credit card. A chemical reaction would then change the color of the card to indicate the possible presence of blood.

Sounds simple enough, but ... some cancers do not bleed on a regular basis, and these would be missed by this test. On the other hand, if you had eaten a cheeseburger or taken an aspirin within several days of the test, there could be a false positive. This means that the test would be positive, but that positive result would not necessarily mean that cancer was present. The test could be falsely positive because taking some medications, such as aspirin, cause some oozing or bleeding from the intestinal tract. And then we have a real problem. Was the bleeding harmless or due to a cancer?

Even if a repeat test is normal, you might have a nagging anxiety that a serious problem could be missed. This is why we don't consistently recommend the fecal occult blood test. If the test is positive, it usually is repeated. If it is positive a second time, then a colonoscopy typically is recommended. If the test is negative, a colonoscopy may still be recommended if you are at high risk for cancer of the colon or rectum (either because of family history or your own history of having multiple polyps in the colon). Many doctors continue to use this test, but only in conjunction with other assessments.

The stool sample test is not a final analysis. Don't rely on it. Your life could hang in the balance.

Sigmoidoscopy

Sigmoidoscopy is not a big deal if the procedure is done by an experienced operator. This screening test is typically done by a primary care physician, an internist (this is not an intern like you see on TV doctor shows, this is a doctor specialized in internal medicine), or a gastroenterologist. To find out how experienced the operator is, ask the doctor how many of these procedures he or she does each year. You want someone who does these all the time.

During the procedure, the doctor inserts a flexible, lighted telescope gently into your rectum and into the lower part of your colon, specifically to search for abnormalities, especially cancer. Patients are often instructed to drink liberal quantities of fluids 24 hours before the procedure and then to use one or two over-the-counter enemas. This consists of a tube, much like a tube of toothpaste, with a small plastic nozzle. The ingredients of the tube are gently squeezed into the rectum to clean out the lining of that organ so the walls of the colon can be clearly seen.

This procedure can be a bit uncomfortable, but, overall, it has relatively few risks and often is safely done on an outpatient basis. Most patients are asked to position themselves in the knee-to-chest position in which they are leaning on their elbows and knees as the tube is inserted. In most cases, IV sedation is not needed. The procedure takes about 15 minutes.

This is an excellent test, but it's not adequate to find a cancer of the colon that may be beyond the reach of the shorter scope. I recommend, instead, a colonoscopy that checks the entire colon.

Colonoscopy

It is not polite dinner conversation to talk about your colonoscopy. However, a colonoscopy, while uncomfortable, is not really a big deal and can give you peace of mind. In other words, don't wait for symptoms. Ask your doctor about setting up a schedule. These aren't the highlight of your year, but they're not a big deal—except when one saves your life.

A colonoscopy usually requires some mild IV sedation, takes about 30 to 45 minutes, and assesses the whole length of the colon. It usually is advocated at age 50 and every 10 years after that, though it may be advised starting earlier in life and more frequently for individuals with polyps or a family history of colon cancer.

Thanks to advancing technology, nearly everything can be "virtual" now, and the colonoscopy is no exception. It's not as simple as we'd like it to be, however. Patients still have to empty their colons with a day of preparation, and if suspicious polyps are spotted on the series of images taken from the outside of the body, guess what's next? A trip inside with a real colonoscope. This is the only way to biopsy any suspicious spots.

Digital rectal examination

Prostate cancer was once viewed as a disease of older men in nursing homes. Not now. For some reason, this cancer has become aggressive and virulent, and it can occur in men in their 40s.

Cancer of the prostate is an enormous problem, especially in the African-American community. The disease seems to occur among younger individuals in this population and may be clinically more dangerous. Interesting studies have suggested that if you're physically active, you may decrease the risk of this cancer.

The digital rectal examination is a routine part of any physical exam. You should expect it to be part of yours. The rectal exam is performed on both men and women. The doctor inserts a lubricated, gloved finger into your rectum. With gentle pressure, an examination in men is done of the lower rectum as well as the prostate. The procedure has virtually no associated risks. For women, the examination is used to detect any masses or abnormalities in the lower rectum.

The digital rectal examination is one attempt to detect a cancer of the rectum at its early stage. If the physician feels an abnormality, this is sometimes followed up with the flexible sigmoidoscopic examination or a colonoscopy. This is an important part of the physical examination, especially if the patient has rectal or anal complaints or concerns.

Sure, it's mildly uncomfortable, but the treatment for an advanced cancer is much rougher to get through. Some patients are examined while they lie on their backs. Others might be asked to fold into the knee-to-chest position while lying on their sides.

As a male, I can understand why patients have little enthusiasm for the digital rectal exam. It is hardly the highlight of my year. When properly done with a fully lubricated and gloved hand, and when not done hastily, the procedure is not a great discomfort. However, I clearly know that cancer of the prostate can be a major-league inconvenience to my retirement plans if not detected early. The exam is rarely painful, takes just a short time (perhaps 30 to 45 seconds), even though it seems like longer. And you get the peace of mind that all is okay.

None of us—men or women—is immune from cancer of the rectum. This is why each of us should expect the annual rectal exam. Less frequently, this exam might detect other potentially serious cancer-related problems. For example, malignant melanoma and skin cancers are sometimes found at the time of the rectal exam. Prior to inserting the gloved and lubricated examining finger, the health care provider should look at the skin between the buttocks and around the anus for telltale signs of a potentially serious problem. Again, these are very rare but curable cancers if detected early. You are much more likely to detect your own skin cancer on an area you look at more often.

Prostate specific antigen (PSA)

The PSA blood test is now being seriously reevaluated and challenged as a routine screening for cancer of the prostate. PSA is a chemical that can be detected in the blood through a simple blood test. Depending on the specific method used, the range of normal may be from 0 up to 4. If the test is higher than 4, that does not necessarily mean that cancer is present. The upper limit of normal gets higher with age.

As men get older, the prostate typically increases in size. The larger the prostate, the higher the normal number can be for the

PSA. However, if the PSA continues to increase, that's when we doctors get concerned that the gland could be harboring a cancer. A doubling of the PSA in a few months is a worrisome sign. As with most medical decisions, care has to be tailored to you.

We now know that African Americans have a strikingly high rate of cancer of the prostate. Therefore, if an African-American man is 42 and his PSA level is 4—with 4 being the upper limit of normal— then additional evaluations need to be made. Generally, the high-risk man might start with a PSA analysis at age 40.

When the level is 4, we closely monitor the situation and worry when it gets to 8 and much higher. Another factor is the rate of increase. In other words, if it takes two or three years for the level to go from 4 to 8, that is much less worrisome than if the level goes from 4 to 8 in a few months. Again, no universal "cookbook" exists, and these laboratory tests can be interpreted only within the context of the individual patient, his age, the rate of increase, family history, and racial and ethnic background.

A biopsy of the prostate normally involves taking multiple samples of tissue from a specific area of abnormality. If we can detect a nodule, or can see a nodule by using ultrasound imaging, we'll get samples from that area of the prostate. However, a very challenging situation is the man who has a rising PSA and a normal gland on physical examination and on ultrasound assessment.

In these situations, the worry is that there are some microscopic cancer cells that cannot be seen or detected, but are clearly present and are producing the elevation of the PSA. In this circumstance some men are advised to undergo biopsies in which samples are randomly taken of the gland. Usually, before the biopsies are obtained, a topical anesthetic is injected into the gland to decrease the discomfort.

Most men tolerate this procedure reasonably well, but there is always concern for blood in the urine and significant discomfort (our way of saying "pain") in a minority of men who undergo biopsies. We take this issue seriously and recognize the risks of multiple biopsies of the prostate. Tissue taken from these samples is examined under a microscope in order to determine if cancer is present.

Most men who already have prostate cancer advocate routine PSA blood testing because they know that early diagnosis will reduce disability and improve quality of life. They've been there and done that, and they want their friends and sons to be vigilant.

This cancer is especially devastating because impotence and incontinence may result—not from the cancer, but from the treatment. Because many men live for years after the diagnosis, quality of life becomes a big issue. We really do not fully understand which men should have their prostates removed as a means of treatment. Some men may have a quiet, smoldering form of the disease for decades. They don't require aggressive treatment. For them, a watch-and-wait approach may be sensible, but the risk is that the cancer could become more serious during this period.

If cancer is present, you should seek another opinion from a specialist in cancer and urology so that you are comfortable making your final decision. Yes, that's *your* decision.

Obviously, no test or exam is foolproof, but a normal rectal exam and a normal PSA are highly reassuring that cancer of the prostate is not present at that time.

And now here's why experts are changing their minds about making this test routine: The PSA used to be viewed as the gold standard to diagnose cancer of the prostate. The thinking went something like this. "The digital rectal examination is a crude assessment of the prostate and if there's an area of thickening, and if the PSA is elevated above normal, that patient would warrant a biopsy. This is common sense." However, life is not simple.

In many circumstances, only a few of the cells viewed under the microscope were actually cancer, and it is difficult to predict if the cells will grow and spread and compromise the life of the patient. In some circumstances these cancerous cells lie dormant and almost never compromise the health of the patient.

But we must recognize that each patient is different. It has been long recognized that African-American men in some circumstances have a more aggressive type of cancer of the prostate, as I've stated. A recent study from Johns Hopkins evaluated African-American men who had what appeared to be low-risk cancer of the prostate. These patients opted for surgery rather than aggressive surveillance. The findings were disturbing. Among these patients with relatively favorable types of cancer of the prostate was a sixfold excess of aggressive cancer cells under the microscope, and these patients were also at higher risk for an elevation of the PSA, which almost always indicates a recurrence of the cancer.

So what is the lesson from this study? We must individualize cancer care; one size does not fit all. In other words, for high-risk populations such as the African-American male, routine surveillance is probably not adequate. These patients need to be aware that more aggressive examinations and possibly imaging studies would be appropriate.

Now let's get back to the general guidelines from responsible medical organizations. The United States Preventive Services Task Force does not recommend routine PSA screening for cancer of the prostate. However, this test is reasonable if patients fall into the following categories: A strong family history of cancer of the prostate, especially occurring at a relatively young age among first-degree relatives (brother, dad); being African-American; a life expectancy of at least 15 more years.

In two landmark studies published in the *New England Journal of Medicine* in 2009, routine screening led to more patients being diagnosed with the disease but no decrease in cancer deaths. This suggests that cancers are being diagnosed at an early stage and in most patients pose little risk to the well-being of that patient. The American Cancer Society suggests a shared decision-making approach and does not support routine testing for a man of average risk. However, knowing the higher risk among individuals with a positive family history for men of African heritage, a frank discussion is appropriate concerning the test and what to do if the results are abnormal.

Bottom line: Some studies indicate that by using the current guidelines, for every 48 men diagnosed with cancer of the prostate through screening and given some form of treatment, only one life was saved. The remaining 47 patients are at risk for obvious complications, such as impotence and incontinence (from surgery), and perhaps these treatments were not indicated since the cancer was not life-threatening.

I know of at least eight men who were faced with this dilemma a decade ago when our knowledge about screening was somewhat primitive. They did undergo radical prostate surgery, and each of them has had some complications.

One of my colleagues was a university professor, and at age 62 he developed symptoms of a urinary tract infection. As part of his evaluation, a routine PSA was obtained. The value was 7, which was nearing the upper limit of normal. The antibiotic treatment cleared the urinary tract infection, but the PSA remained elevated. A careful digital rectal examination suggested some thickening of the prostate, so a biopsy was recommended.

Approximately 10 percent of the biopsy specimen identified obvious malignant/cancerous cells, meaning that 90 percent of the specimen was not malignant. You can imagine the dilemma this patient and his physician now faced.

Of course, this scenario took place about 10 years ago, before there was a clear understanding of the fact that some of these cancers almost never spread. Our patient was advised to have surgery, so he underwent a radical procedure to remove the prostate and the surrounding tissue. It was a great feeling of relief when the cancer was confined to the prostate, and there was the expectation of a cure. That was the good news. Here's the bad news. Impotence was an issue, incontinence was an embarrassing dilemma, and the patient's quality of life—especially as a visible professional—was profoundly compromised.

If this scenario played out today, we may have taken a different approach. Without a doubt, there would've been a heartfelt discussion with the patient, and, if appropriate, with the spouse or partner, concerning what the next steps would be.

So what can each of us take away from this thorny issue of prostate cancer screening?

We need to do our homework. We need to recognize that medicine is a science, but it is also certainly an art. If the gentleman is, let's say, in his early 70s, with a youthful and vital lifestyle, and let's say his spouse or partner is 40 years of age, our patient may opt for aggressive surveillance rather than risking the life-altering consequences of treatment.

All the facts and figures in the literature become somewhat of an interesting academic exercise until it's *your* PSA and *your* prostate. Then the stakes become clear.

Enter the empowered patient. A survey of men ages 40 to 74 found that 54 percent said they would still want a PSA test, despite the recommendations and risks. And a University of Texas study found that more than 40 percent of men over age 75 still undergo PSA screening because their primary care docs are continuing the practice.

Bottom line: Although controversy exists among the experts, the weight of evidence and the standard of medical practice in most communities is for the digital rectal examination and the PSA to be performed annually, or more frequently, based on the patient's age and risks for either cancer of the prostate or cancer of the rectum. But there needs to be a frank discussion. *Okay, if we get the PSA and it is elevated, then what do we do?*

Now a word about a cancer that men don't talk about. Testicular cancer is the most common cancer in men between ages 20 and 34. That is why each testicle needs to be examined during the physical. Every man should examine his own testicles monthly anyway. Don't ignore a painless mass or an aching discomfort in the scrotum or groin. If you have an area of concern, a testicular ultrasound may be done. This involves placing a small device (it looks like a microphone) on the testicle. The ultrasound images are then reviewed for cancerous masses or areas of suspicion.

Pap test and pelvic examination

All women who are, or have been, sexually active or have reached age 18 should have an annual Pap test and pelvic examination. After a woman has had three or more consecutive satisfactory normal annual examinations, the Pap test may be performed less frequently at the discretion of the physician. And after a discussion with the patient.

Cancer of the cervix is a preventable and curable cancer, if detected early. With positive lymph nodes, meaning the cancer has spread, the chance of cure decreases dramatically—often vanishing. The treatment often involves a combination of chemotherapy and radiation. The routine Pap smear is the best way to eliminate the difficult treatment required by this type of tumor.

Expect a Pap test and pelvic examination as part of your annual checkup. During the Pap test, a small brush is inserted into the opening of the uterus. Cells are scraped off, placed on a glass slide or into a small bottle, and looked at under a microscope. As part of the procedure, a physical exam is done of the female organs and rectum.

At one time, a woman would undergo a routine Pap smear and pelvic exam every year, regardless of her age. It is now becoming clear that as individuals reach their 70s and 80s, this recommendation needs to be reevaluated. If a woman is not sexually active and has had no previously abnormal Pap smears, to discontinue the annual Pap smear in the 70s certainly seems reasonable.

But again, many of these recommendations need to be applied to each specific patient. For example, if a woman in her 30s has multiple sexual partners and is sexually active, yearly Pap smears and pelvic exams are certainly appropriate. On the other hand, if a woman is celibate and does not have any significant gynecologic history, performing Pap smears and pelvic exams at a less frequent interval certainly makes good sense.

Older women should be alert to the significance of bleeding from the uterus after menopause. A cancer of the uterus may first become evident by bleeding from the vagina. Again, early detection gives far better odds of a cure than detecting a cancer that has spread. In most cases, bleeding is not serious. But if it continues, it does need attention. Expect your doctor to recommend an endometrial tissue sample (biopsy), especially if you experience postmenopausal bleeding. And be certain to ask for a copy of the pathology report so there is no misunderstanding of what was seen under the microscope.

A scraping of the lining of the uterus (for an endometrial uterine biopsy) is an office procedure with low risks. Occasionally, cancer cells from the ovary may be detected this way. Again, early detection raises the odds of long-term cure. Don't ignore your body's signals that something's wrong.

A vaccine to protect against cervical cancer is now available for a whole generation of young women. It is particularly important in underserved populations in this country and throughout the world for whom cervical cancer unfortunately remains a leading cause of death. The vaccine against cancer shows the value of tenacious research. Because some cervical cancers develop from exposure to the human papillomavirus (often a sexually transmitted disease), this may be a model for attacking some other virus-triggered cancers, but a vaccine is not yet applicable to the big killers: lung, breast, colon, and prostate cancers.

Breast self-exam

As every woman reading this book knows, breast cancer is a national catastrophe. Approximately one woman in eight or nine will develop this cancer. The emotional and psychological impact of breast cancer is profound. Spectacular advances in the hormonal treatment of breast cancer have opened great possibilities for long-term benefit. However, we need to recognize that, as with colon cancer, early detection is the key.

Every woman knows these self-exams aren't foolproof, but we all know you need to do it every month. Some studies have suggested that the breast self-exam is not necessary. In fact, headlines such as "Study finds no evidence that teaching breast self-examination saves lives" make me cringe. A study in the *Journal of the National Cancer Institute* found that women who examined their breasts found lumps that turned out to be fine after a small surgical procedure. The bottom line for the researchers was that these unnecessary biopsies added to already high health care costs.

The researchers also concluded that doctors should not spend time teaching women how to conduct a breast self-exam, but should spend more time educating women about breast cancer symptoms, such as a lump or nipple discharge, and should also spend more time on the clinical breast exam they conduct in the office.

I think a woman should be proactive and assertive in asking for instructions on breast self-exam. We are clearly learning that the physical exam alone is not adequate to detect cancers, so this technique must be used in concert with mammograms.

A revealing survey by the Susan G. Komen Breast Cancer Foundation found that young women in their 20s and 30s are not performing monthly breast self-exams because most don't think they are at risk. Certainly being a woman and growing older are risk factors, but breast cancer remains the leading cause of cancer for women in this younger age range too. Sadly, women diagnosed this young often have a more aggressive form of the disease.

Mammography

Mammograms can detect a cancer the size of a grain of rice and can offer a high chance of cure. My female patients tell me the anticipation of having a mammogram creates an enormous amount of anxiety. The area of the clinic where the mammograms are done is one of the most tense pieces of real estate in a medical institution. The reason is obvious.

Every woman knows what the radiologist is looking for, and every woman dreads the possibility of a malignant tumor being detected in her breast. I almost always ask patients about the level of discomfort from the procedure. In general, I am hearing that the discomfort largely depends on the skill and the sensitivity of the technician performing the test. And the discomfort does not seem to correlate with the age of the patient or the breast size.

For reasons that I do not think that any of us really understands, the procedure can go smoothly in some women without much discomfort, but in others it can be uncomfortable. The size and contour of the breasts does not seem to make a difference in comfort level. One factor makes the test somewhat bearable. The discomfort only lasts for a few moments, and most patients are able to understand the importance of "bearing with" the compression of the breasts while the test is performed.

Although some controversy exists regarding the schedule for screening mammograms, the American Cancer Society now recommends starting with a mammogram at age 40, then every year through age 70 or 75, and even later. Women should have an annual mammogram in conjunction with a clinical breast examination. In this procedure, your doctor will carefully examine each breast and palpate (or feel) the tissue as you sit, again while you lie down, and also as you stand with your hands on your hips. He or she will pay careful attention to the lymph nodes in the areas behind the collarbone and in the armpit.

Here's why the lymph nodes are so important. The larger the cancer, the greater chance the lymph nodes are contaminated. If the breast cancer is detected early, it is highly curable. With lymph nodes involved, chances for cure drop. And cure chances also drop with larger-sized cancer.

If the cancer is small (an inch or less), then cure rates at 20 years may be almost 90 percent. But if the cancer is 4 inches or larger, the average time for the cancer to come back may be months, and almost none are cured. Even one involved lymph node dramatically reduces the chances for cure. For patients with 1 to 3 nodes involved, the 10-year survival rate is about 50 percent.

As of this writing, a study in the *British Medical Journal* has cast some doubt on whether regular mammograms save lives. Until their findings are carefully scrutinized, and possible recommendations amended, let's go with what we know, and I know that early detection saves lives. That message is especially compelling when that life is your mother, your sister, your daughter, or yourself.

Don't rely on the "system" to send you reminder notices about your next mammogram. It's up to you to remember when you had a mammogram and to schedule another in about a year. Absolutely begin screening with these simple X-rays by age 40. A clinical breast examination is done by a doctor or nurse-practitioner.

Men, too, can get breast cancer. (However, women never get prostate cancer!) A painless lump or nipple discharge needs to be assessed with a mammogram and a careful physical exam. A biopsy is often done to determine the diagnosis. About 30 percent of these men have a positive family history of breast cancer in either males or females. That's why doctors should ask about your family tree.

Health counseling and cancer checkup

We know good habits must be formed and reinforced early. That's why the American Cancer Society recommends a cancer checkup and health counseling every 3 years, starting as young as age 20, and then annually after age 40.

Now here's what a doctor is looking for in examining the rest of your body in these annual (and sort-of-annual) physicals:

Thyroid: If your thyroid gland (at the bottom of your neck, in front) is enlarged, a simple biopsy with a needle can determine if a cancer is present. This is usually preceded by an ultrasound evaluation, which consists of placing a microphone-type device over the base of the neck near the Adam's apple. With early detection, you have a high chance for cure.

Lymph nodes: If they are enlarged, it could mean lymphoma or Hodgkin's disease (cancers of the lymph nodes or bone marrow). But most swollen nodes are not cancerous.

Mouth: Simple inspection of your tongue, palate, lips, and cheeks (inside) can detect an early and curable cancer. Dental hygienists perform this routinely while cleaning your teeth. They are the first to spot oral cancers, especially among smokers and those who chew tobacco.

Skin: There are specific ways to tell if a mole is malignant once it is found—by you or your physician. If it is removed early, the chance of a cure is virtually assured. If not found early, you may face major surgery and possibly need aggressive chemotherapy with or without radiation.

When Screening Is Not Enough—The Lungs

When it comes to lung cancer, there's no mystery. What a national and global catastrophe! Lung cancer is the number 1 cause of cancer-related deaths in men and women. It accounts for one-third of all cancer deaths. And it is preventable, because smoking is the "smoking gun" in almost all cases.

The progression is simple: The younger the age you start to smoke, and the more cigarettes you smoke over your soon-to-be-abbreviated lifetime, the greater your risk. But it is never too late to stop. Studies show that after a number of years without smoking, the risk of lung cancer decreases, and, eventually, your risk approaches that of a nonsmoker.

By the time a chest X-ray shows lung cancer, it has been present for at least four to six years and contains a billion cancer cells. So early detection really does not apply to lung cancer, and you can't rely on a chest X-ray. Fortunately, early work with the spiral CT scan may show lung cancers earlier, and we now have evidence that screening selected smokers in this manner will catch lung cancers earlier and lower the death rate.

So how do we normally detect lung cancer? Our patients typically show up coughing bloody phlegm, with shortness of breath, pneumonia, weight loss, bone pain, hoarseness, and shoulder or arm pain. And if the cancer has already spread to the brain—because lung cancer is highly aggressive—a patient may feel weakness in an arm or leg, suffer confusion, and have headaches or seizures.

Few advanced lung cancer patients live longer than a year. But miracles do indeed happen. One of my patients had a highly aggressive and virulent form of lung cancer, which, with treatment, was moved away from major structures around the heart and aorta. He had a stormy postoperative course but has made a full recovery.

The madness about cancer is that we have the tools, techniques, and education to dramatically enhance the health, wellness, and quality of life for ourselves, family, friends, and neighbors. We need to be proactive, assertive, and informed—and we need to take charge.

Are You Ever Too Old for Screening?

Doctors can agree on when to start health screening, such as routine mammograms, but we can't agree on when to stop screening. Some doctors think age 75 may signal the end of routine screenings for breast, colon, and cervical cancer. After all, they reason, an older person may suffer more harm from a false positive and surgery. A 90-year-old man with a small prostate tumor will die from something else, not prostate cancer. They see no economic benefit in terms of years of life saved (of course, they're not talking about your father). But I continue to care for patients in their 80s who look 50, are vital and active, and in these patients we really need to offer selected screening tools.

Now comes the tension between experts caring for the individual patient and experts responsible for national health policy. A middle road exists: Each patient needs to be viewed as an individual, not as a cold statistic or a blip on some economist's spreadsheet.

We need to acknowledge that we are living longer than any generation in history (for a good reason), and if a woman is married and 65, she may well live to be over 90 years old. Now if the screening test is painful, difficult to prepare for (as some think preparing for a colonoscopy is difficult), and if the patient has no complaints and a negative family history, then fine. Forgo the procedure. But mammograms in a woman who may live to 100 do not seem unreasonable.

Think about it. People are living longer because we're screening and catching the high blood pressure, the precancerous lesion, the elevated blood glucose, the tiny skin cancer—or I'd sure like to think so.

But this decision is yours. As a general rule, if you have an anticipated life expectancy of 10 more years, continuing your annual screening may be a reasonable choice.

Who Is Best at Detecting Skin Cancer?

Generally, you, not your doctor or a nurse, are the first to detect a malignant melanoma (a deadly form of skin cancer) when it occurs on your skin. Not surprisingly, women more frequently detect a malignant melanoma than do men. This is consistent with many studies documenting that women are the drivers of health care consumerism, and it is the woman who often makes health care decisions for the entire family.

So don't wait for an annual physical exam to see if the doctor spies something unusual. If you think a mole looks different in some way or a freckle is changing, see your doctor right away. When it comes to your family, it sure doesn't hurt to give each other a once-over. Here's why.

In about 10 to 15 percent of people with malignant melanoma, the first indication of a problem arises from the metastatic disease (the spread of cancer from one organ to another) rather than from the primary, or what is known as the "occult primary site." Let me explain.

A fairly common scenario is that a person awakens one day and finds a lump under the armpit or in the groin. A biopsy of the lymph node shows malignant melanoma. In around 90 percent of people, a primary malignant melanoma can be detected in the vicinity of the armpit or near the groin. This was the "mother cancer" from whence arises the rogue cell that seeds into the lymph nodes. These primary sites are what we all want to detect early—long before the cancer decides to move anywhere else in your body.

But in the other 10 percent of people, we never find the primary neoplasm (or mole). We suspect that there was a primary at some point in time, but then the primary dries up, falls off, or is somehow devoured by the body's immune system. However, this process does not occur until after a bizarre cell has broken loose from the primary site and set up a beachhead in a lymph node.

A swollen lymph node may not be the first sign. In some people, the first evidence of malignant melanoma is a seizure. An appropriate scan of the brain then documents metastatic malignant melanoma, but a primary site is never found. At this point, finding the primary site is not relevant. The patient is faced with a far-advanced disease somewhere else, such as the brain, bone, liver, or spinal cord.

Here are some other examples of what we call the "unknown primary malignant melanoma" that we see on a fairly consistent basis:

- A woman who has a routine Pap smear and pelvic exam shows evidence of a vaginal/rectal malignant melanoma. This obviously is not an area exposed to the sun, and so it does emphasize how little we really do understand about these tumors.

- An individual has a lump under the skin that seems to be innocent, but a biopsy (tissue sample) shows malignant melanoma.
- Someone who coughs up blood has a chest X-ray that is abnormal. A biopsy of the lung indicates metastatic malignant melanoma in the lungs, without any obvious primary site.

In other words, a lump or bump or a spot or a swelling that is relatively new and without obvious explanation (you don't remember hitting it accidentally or falling and being injured) certainly could be a metastatic deposit of malignant melanoma, even when the primary malignant melanoma is not detected.

Have I made my point about screening? About knowing your body and knowing when something is different? A few minutes in front of the mirror may be the cheapest medical test you'll ever have. The comments from spouse or partner about the skin are crucial, especially for moles on the back.

Other Screening Tests: Well Worth Paying For or Not Worth the Time and Money?

You may have heard about certain screening tests other than the standard tests recommended by the American Cancer Society and American Heart Association. Some of these can be useful in certain circumstances, depending on your family history. Some of them may well be worth paying for (because your insurance company may not cover them). Others may not be a good investment of your time and money. But let's look at some options.

Genetic testing for diseases

Some families are at an especially high risk for cancers arising from the colon and rectum, or for Huntington's and other genetic diseases, or for the BRCA breast cancer genes. If you have a first-degree relative (mother, father, brother, sister) who has had this disease, or if there are family members with disease occurring at relatively young ages (younger than 40), you may be at risk.

Genetic tests can be performed on your blood to identify abnormalities in genetic material which might signal that you're prone to developing the disease. However, as with most tests and medicine, the findings are not absolutely foolproof. Sometimes the results can be misleading. And detecting an abnormal gene in your DNA does not necessarily mean that you will develop something.

There is another problem: You can imagine the psychological impact of being told that you have a defective gene and that you might develop cancer of the colon, for example. That's the dark side to genetic testing. If a genetic test is "positive" and that leaves you at risk for developing a disease, what does this mean for your employability and insurability? Would you miss out on a job because your employer finds out you may be at risk? The answer is not clear, and we could spend lots of emotional energy to sort this out. We can make better use of our time.

So what are some practical suggestions?

Genetic testing is a highly personal decision. Some people have a need to know, and if that is your situation, a blood test would be reasonable as long as you fully recognize the limitations of that test. From a practical standpoint, screening colonoscopy starting at age 40, or 10 years before the youngest member of the family developed colon cancer, would be smart.

Testing for endometrial and ovarian cancers

If you're a woman beyond menopause and you have vaginal bleeding, then your doctor may discuss with you a scraping of the lining of the uterus. This material is then looked at under the microscope to see if it contains cancer. This procedure, an endometrial or uterine biopsy, is typically performed in the doctor's office. It's relatively safe and is an important test to discuss with your doctor.

A transvaginal ultrasound consists of a small probe somewhat like a thermometer being inserted into the vagina. The probe is then gently positioned through the cervix, which is the opening leading into the uterus itself. This is an outpatient/office procedure and typically is not any more uncomfortable than having a routine Pap smear and pelvic examination—so my female patients tell me.

The images obtained from the ultrasound can help determine if there are masses or abnormalities in the pelvic area. These images are not photographs but look like a weather map. As with many imaging interventions, this test likewise is not foolproof. But if a woman has symptoms, such as pain, bloating, or fullness, and if there is a family history of female cancers, this test is reasonable.

CA-125 (the CA stands for carbohydrate antigen) is a substance found in blood that acts as a marker or a barometer or a "surrogate" for some types of cancers. It was thought that an elevated CA-125 level might indicate that a woman had ovarian cancer. However, the test is not perfect and is not always specific for cancer. Some women may have an elevated CA-125 but may not have a malignant disease. But the test is still used, along with scans and a physical exam, to monitor whether chemotherapy is working to contain certain female cancers.

Now what about getting the CA-125 "just to make certain that everything is okay"? The problem with this approach is that the levels may be minimally elevated, and CT scans or ultrasound examinations of the abdomen and pelvis may not confirm or rule out that a cancer exists. Then what do you do? We can imagine the anxiety of this situation. Therefore, if you do not have specific symptoms and if your family history is not overwhelmingly positive, these types of tests are not routinely done.

Early mammograms for breast cancer

One thing is clear, mammograms are detecting breast cancers at a far more curable stage than at any time in history. It is not uncommon to see breast cancers that are about the size of a match head being detected on the mammogram.

But when mammograms are performed in women younger than 40, the results are sometimes difficult to interpret. Younger women's breasts are normally dense, and the mammograms are not as reliable as they are for older women. With age, the density becomes less intense, and fat becomes more apparent on the mammogram. The contrast between the fat in the breast tissue and the normal breast glands allows for more accurate detection of significant abnormalities.

Generally, though, most professional medical groups agree that a yearly mammogram should be performed, starting at age 40.

Genetic mutation–linked cancers (BRCA1, BRCA2)

Within the last decade, scientists identified genes BRCA1 and BRCA2 which, when normal, facilitate the repair of DNA. This protects against the development of cancer. On the other hand, when these genes are abnormal or defective, risk of cancer is strikingly higher. Some studies suggest that when these genes are abnormal, women may have a 56 to 87 percent lifetime chance of developing breast cancer and a 20 to 60 percent chance of developing ovarian cancer.

As with other forms of genetic testing, the analysis of chromosomes for these defective genes has far-reaching implications. Here is the dilemma: "If I as a woman have an abnormal gene, does this mean my other family members should be tested? Even if my gene is abnormal, I may not necessarily develop breast cancer, but my risks are high."

If a woman is at high risk for these cancers because she has many first-degree family members having this condition, genetic testing is reasonable. But I suggest you need to ask a piercing question first: *If I test abnormal, what do I do with the results?*

In this case, some women, in order to give themselves the best chance of long-term survival, have opted to have both breasts removed, and some patients are advised to have their ovaries removed as well. Studies now demonstrate that this is a reasonable option for some women who are especially concerned about the probability of developing breast cancer. And if the ovaries are removed, this eliminates the risks for ovarian cancer, but these are obviously major operations.

As another option, if the test is positive, a woman can work with her doctor to develop a plan for careful surveillance in terms of yearly mammograms, prompt biopsies of suspicious lumps or bumps, ovarian surveillance, and the importance of both a professional breast exam and careful training in breast self-exams.

The shopping-center full-body scan

Technology can be a wondrous thing. Or not. Or maybe?

It is now becoming fashionable for companies to set up in shopping centers with mobile PET scanners and mobile CT scanners and mobile MRI scanners. These are marvelous high-tech imaging techniques that can detect problems long before they become significant or meaningful. And that's the problem.

Let's suppose we scan 100 individuals. Almost all of them, if they are adults, will have some spots and shadows on their lungs, for example, which almost never turn out to be cancer. But once we know "something is there," these suspicious areas will need to be followed up, and that means more expensive tests, more anxiety, and more inconvenience for the patient. With a high-tech scan, the "worried well" have opened up Pandora's box and will never be able to get it closed again.

The scanners can see abnormalities, but they can't tell us what they are. So at some point, the patient may become increasingly uneasy about these spots, and a major operation may be necessary to check it out. Mayo Clinic studies and other institutions have documented that patients may undergo extensive surgery, which obviously is life-threatening, to remove some harmless spots that never would have caused problems.

Therefore, we need ongoing studies to really determine if these shopping-center scans are of any value, or if they are simply detecting problems that would never pose any threat to the individual. Worse yet, someone who undergoes a scan and comes out fine may be tempted to skip a regular physical exam for blood pressure testing, cholesterol levels, and other key blood work that the scans don't evaluate.

Our current system of screening works. However, high-tech scans are not always helpful and can be harmful, especially for relatively healthy people who have no symptoms. If you decide to undergo extensive, additional high-tech scans, you will want to decide up front what you will do about those shadows and spots, if any are detected. Surely, you seek a "clean bill of health," but as we become more sophisticated in peeking inside the human body, we have the unfortunate ability to create more anxiety about the unknown.

Let's Get Physical

The executive physical—it's a highly prized perk for corporate execs, but you can have one too, even if you don't run General Motors. I've asked my colleagues to explain the real "ins and outs" of the popular executive physical conducted at the clinic. I talked with Dr. Philip T. Hagen and Dr. Donald D. Hensrud in the Department of Preventive Medicine.

Among the CEO crowd, appointment times for these physicals are scheduled a year ahead. But you don't have to wait. You can get the same high-level care from your doctor if you know what to ask for and insist that your doctor partner with you in your care.

Your medical history

The medical history (which includes your family health history) generally begins with questions like this:
- How are things going?
- How are you feeling?
- What is it that concerns you the most?
- What are you worried about?
- What brings you to see us today?

I've come to realize that it's the second or third concern the patient mentions, in some circumstances, that is the most significant one. It's my experience that patients don't always know which of their complaints is the most serious. I may be much more concerned about a patient who casually mentions sudden headaches than about the weight gain that causes them the greatest distress.

Bring a list of all medications you are taking, including prescription drugs, vitamins, minerals, herbs, supplements, nasal sprays, patches, creams, ointments—everything. Know the dose of everything you are taking and how often you take it. And also know who advised you to start these medications. Sometimes it's easier to dump all your medications in a bag and bring them with you. The smart strategy, however, is to keep a written record on a file card and keep this card with you (in a wallet or purse) at all times.

Now you can find apps to track your medications; you can download these for your smartphone or tablet. Such a practice could be lifesaving if you find yourself in a real-life episode of *Grey's Anatomy* or *House*. I've also seen apps to help patients manage their type 2 diabetes using their mobile phones, and preliminary results are finding patients lowering their overall blood sugars.

Any medication can produce *side effects*, which are undesirable results from ingredients in the medication. Some are tolerable, such as dry mouth, or unacceptable, such as increased liver damage or heart palpitations. *Interactions*, on the other hand, occur when two or more active ingredients in substances you are taking affect each other. It's the interaction effect that concerns doctors and pharmacists, such as when patients mix prescription drugs and herbals, for example. Herbals can increase or decrease the effects of some medications when used together. At highest risk for interactions are people with chronic conditions, such as stroke, high blood pressure, diabetes, and heart disease. Your physical exam may be an ideal time to discuss if you even need to continue taking certain medications.

If you're presenting certain symptoms when you visit the doctor, it will be important for the doctor to rule out or rule in interactions as causes. Even substances you might consider harmless can cause problems, so let your doctor know about *everything* you're taking. Here are two examples:

- Some forms of ginseng may interfere with a blood thinner you are taking to prevent stroke. It also lowers blood sugar in people who take medicine for diabetes. Even ginseng tea can cause drug-herbal interactions.
- Garlic supplements can change the results of your blood-clotting tests. People who take arthritis pain medications may also be at risk for bruising by taking garlic. And garlic may increase the effect of blood sugar–lowering drugs for those who take diabetes medications. Garlic cooked in foods becomes inactivated because of the heat, so it's fine. Interactions can occur with fresh garlic and concentrated supplements.
- Grapefruit, believe it or not, can make some drugs you take more potent. Some of these include certain drugs for lowering cholesterol. If you eat grapefruit or drink the juice,

ask your doctor (better yet, your pharmacist) if any of the

drugs you take interact with grapefruit or other citrus fruits.

It's also important to fill the doctor in on what you do for a living, your travels, your hobbies, your social ties, where you live and have lived in the past, and your family responsibilities. Everything you say (whether the doctor asks you directly or not) gives the doctor a picture of you.

I recently had the opportunity of seeing a woman who had a stressful job in a high-tech company. She took an early buy-out and had a wonderful first and second year of retirement. She and her husband then bought into a family-run business—and the nightmare began. Following a contentious interchange with some unpleasant family members, our patient developed crushing chest pain that lasted for two hours. She was rushed to the hospital, and underwent a complete battery of cardiac assessments that indicated no muscle damage but clearly showed that stress caused the chest problem. Life pressures like this are why your doctor really needs to know your social and occupational situation.

Here's another example. A charming 82-year-old grandmother finally admitted she was having chest pain after three days of discomfort. She called her doctor, who directed her to the emergency room. On day 3 in the hospital, and after many tests, the doctors felt she was fine to return home. They increased her heart medication. But it wasn't until her daughter-in-law collared one of the attending physicians in the hospital hallway, asking him, "Did she mention that her grandson was getting a divorce and that's been bothering her?" that they put all the pieces together.

The doctors had been busy conducting sophisticated stress tests and medical procedures and had not looked at the whole person. If they had, they would have seen a dear woman whose heart literally ached. When the initial medical history was taken in the ER, she, of course, had not mentioned her family distress. Had the doctor asked or had she thought it relevant, such information would have been a key point in her medical history. A key question for us providers: Can you tell me about yourself? I need to know who you are and what you now do or have done for a living.

Your family history is also crucial for the doctor to know. We should each have a general understanding of the health of our relatives, and that includes mother, father, aunts and uncles, and of course brothers and sisters. This is especially relevant for heart disease, certain neurologic disorders, allergies, and certainly for cancer.

At the end of the medical history taking or at the end of the consultation, you should have a feeling of closure and validation. Have your issues been addressed courteously and professionally? If not, speak up!

Your physical examination

This typically follows the taking of the medical history. Up to this point, I hope you have been sitting comfortably either in an exam room chair or in the doctor's personal office, having a face-to-face discussion without distractions. With all your clothes on. And the provider has looked at you and not just at the computer screen. For me the electronic tablet is magical. I have all the clinical data on the glass screen and can face the patient as we talk.

In most circumstances, at least for a general medical examination or for your first visit, you will eventually be asked to disrobe completely. You will be asked to wear a paper or cloth gown, which may or may not have sleeves. The doctor's staff will take and note your vital signs. This consists of your pulse, temperature, weight, and blood pressure.

Following a washing of the hands as a symbolic way of starting the physical exam, the doctor will listen to your heart and lungs through a stethoscope, and will typically feel around your neck, under your arms, on your breasts and abdomen, and in your rectum, and also carefully examine your skin throughout the whole process. The doctor also may place the stethoscope on your neck to hear your carotid arteries. These main blood vessels supply blood and life-sustaining oxygen to your brain. A blockage here can lead to stroke and death. If there is a characteristic noise in the carotid, called a bruit, this might reflect a decreased blood supply (think blockage here), and then your doctor may recommend a more sophisticated test with an ultrasound.

The knees and ankles typically are tapped with a reflex hammer. The doctor will use a lighted instrument to examine your eyes, mouth, nose, and ears.

The physical exam should not be painful, but it can be somewhat embarrassing and rather uncomfortable as your abdomen is prodded or your rectum examined. The occurrence of sexually transmitted diseases can be detected by the history and physical examination.

Usually, the history taking would take about 10 to 15 minutes, based on the complexity of your case, and the physical exam an equal amount of time. If your doctor has slotted 10 minutes for your first exam, there simply won't be enough time, so when you make your appointment, make sure to ask for adequate time. Otherwise, you may have to return to continue the history and physical. And that's not fair to you. If the doctor is called away to an emergency and makes an exit during the exam, reschedule. You should feel you are being listened to respectfully.

Top 10 Symptoms Not to Ignore (So Don't Wait until Your Next Physical Exam)

1. **Fatigue** of more than one week's duration without obvious explanation: If you have the flu or are recovering from a surgery or accident, feeling tired is normal. However, hoist the red flags if you're tired for no obvious reason, if you find yourself running out of steam in the early to midafternoon, if you push yourself during the week only to collapse in a heap on the weekend, or if you become listless and indifferent to your normal responsibilities. Fatigue usually does not represent a significant problem, but if it lasts more than a week and there are no obvious explanations, see your doctor.

2. **Cough:** We all cough. That is just the nature of the lives we live. A cough that lasts more than 5 to 10 days, especially if you are a smoker and particularly if you

start coughing up thick green or ropy phlegm or have blood in your phlegm, is something to be concerned about. And I'm talking about lung cancer. Shortness of breath and weight loss associated with a cough are serious. We need to also think about TB (tuberculosis), depending upon where the patient lives (or has lived). See your doctor right away.

3. **Pain:** As we get older, we all have aches and pains. Almost always these are not significant. But if pain lasts more than three to five days in a specific area without obvious explanation, you should have it checked out. Obviously, if you have fallen and hurt your shoulder or banged your knee on the bedpost, you'll have pain. But any pain that comes out of nowhere, that awakens you at night, and that clearly does not improve should be checked.

4. **Chest pain:** Here's the big one many men and women foolishly ignore. Chest pain that occurs if you exert yourself, and chest pain that might be described as a squeezing or heavy feeling in your chest, could indicate a heart attack. If the pain extends into your jaw or left shoulder, you are toying with disaster. Don't wait for all these symptoms to appear or disappear. Get emergency care *now.*

5. **Blood:** Blood in the rectum, stool, urine, or phlegm is a signal. With a vigorous wiping of the rectal/anal area, it is not surprising that the toilet paper might have a pink tinge. Almost never is this a cause for alarm. However, if there is obvious blood on the stool (take a look), and if there is pain with passing a bowel movement, this usually is caused by hemorrhoids. These are prominent blood vessels around the anal opening, much like a small group of grapes. Here's the fatal pitfall. It is easy to think the blood from your rectum may be caused by hemorrhoids, when in fact you may have an underlying cancer. That's why, especially in adults, this symptom

should not be ignored. If you have a family history of colorectal cancer, all the more reason to see your doctor and check the source of the blood.

6. **A new lump or bump:** This means a lump or bump that is not particularly painful, and one that has not been associated with trauma. Cancer usually is not painful. A lump or bump that has occurred relatively quickly and feels tender is almost always not a cancer. But if it doesn't disappear over a week or so and you can't remember if you hurt yourself there, a professional evaluation would be important. And you might expect a biopsy to remove the bump and have it looked at under the microscope.

7. **Moles:** Malignant melanoma is one of the most rapidly increasing cancers. If a mole rapidly appears or darkens or itches over a relatively short number of months, or starts to bleed, you need to have a biopsy (cells are then viewed under a microscope).

8. **Weight loss:** As a society, we are consumed with diets. Don't think so? Check out the tabloids as you go through the checkout line in the supermarket. But weight loss without a diet is another matter. Many people who experience a dramatic loss of weight might dance in the street. Some of us pay a lot of money for diet plans to do just that. But a relatively quick loss of weight—faster than 2 or 3 pounds a week—may signal an underlying problem, such as a thyroid gland that needs to be addressed. Weight loss is commonly a concern if you lose 10 percent of your body weight over a three-month period, yet you haven't changed your eating habits or increased your physical activity.

9. **Headaches:** We all get headaches. We live in a tense society. Headaches often are related to tension and stress and rarely are brain tumors, although that can be your first thought. Don't ignore the relatively new onset of a new

type of headache, especially if it occurs in the morning and increases when you cough or sneeze, because that combination could signal a serious condition.

10. **Stroke signs:** Weakness of an arm or a leg, or numbness and tingling of an arm, leg, the face or tongue, or difficulty with speech, could indicate the potential onset of a stroke. A stroke causes the death of brain tissue because the blood supply to certain parts of your brain is interrupted. This is a 911 emergency. Don't wait for symptoms to go away, because sometimes these mini-strokes or transient ischemic attacks (TIAs) return in the "big one." And you may not survive that stroke.

I find that many patients cannot be expected to accurately describe many of these symptoms. Often, our patients might say, "Doc, I just don't feel right. I feel lousy." You cannot know if these are a big deal, a little deal, or a minor nuisance. At this point in an office visit, the careful physician will encourage you to elaborate on how you're feeling, and then with insight, professionalism, and judgment, the physician can outline the most appropriate tests to home in on your problem.

Routine testing

Someone going through an executive health program would have all these routine tests performed. You might expect these too:

- **Complete blood count (CBC):** The doctor may ask a medical assistant to draw one or two vials of blood from a vein in your arm. This blood is sent to a laboratory, and the results are reported back to the doctor who will discuss the results with you. The complete blood count basically looks for evidence of anemia (low red blood cell count) and measures the infection-fighting white blood cells, as well as immune-related cells, and cells related to blood clotting, which are called platelets.

- **Glucose:** This is a test for blood sugar (also determined from a sample of your blood). If you are asked to fast before your blood is drawn at your appointment, don't eat for six to eight hours. Usually, black coffee without cream is allowed, as are unlimited fluids, such as water. High blood sugar levels may mean diabetes or prediabetes, and further testing may be done.

- **Blood chemistries:** The blood chemistries measure the balance of your body minerals, as well as how well your liver and kidneys are working. It's amazing what we can tell from blood. These are generic, off-the-shelf screening studies. If any of these measures are abnormal (too high or too low), your doctor will follow up with additional tests.

- **Lipid screen:** This is a barometer of fitness and might also indicate the potential role of weight reduction, physical activity, or the use of medication. Many people know their total cholesterol level and can have this screened at a drugstore, worksite, or community health fair. But the overall measures of the kinds of cholesterol (both good HDL and bad LDL), along with triglycerides, give a better picture of your heart health and potential risk for heart disease.

- **Iron:** If you are having a first-time physical, the doctor may also check your serum iron and iron-binding capacity because this would help screen for disorders of iron metabolism, such as hemochromatosis—a condition in which you have too much iron in your blood. This is treatable, but we need to know about it.

- **Other blood tests** may be ordered to look at how well your thyroid is working, to rule out certain sexually transmitted diseases, a blood level for certain medications whose effects are determined by the amount of the substance in your bloodstream, and any number of other measures your doctor may be checking.

- **Urinalysis:** The urinalysis looks for evidence of red blood cells, infection, or protein in a sample of your urine. If blood is present in the sample, you may need additional tests. If protein is present to a significant degree, this could indicate kidney disease.

- **Nutrition assessment:** Usually, if a patient is generally healthy, there is no need for a nutrition class, but if a patient has kidney disease or certain intestinal diseases, such as sprue or celiac disease or colitis, there might be a role for consultation with a dietitian. These patients may need and welcome recommendations on dietary and nutritional issues.

  If there are significant cardiac or diabetic concerns, then referral to specialists may be appropriate. Patients usually are asked to fill out a food diary, which outlines what they eat over several typical days. Dietitians are sub-specialized much like medical care providers. In the Mayo Clinic program, our patients may meet with a dietitian for heart disease, renal (kidney) disease, or intestinal diseases, or to specifically focus on diabetes. Your doctor may refer you to a specialist in your community, or you can locate a qualified dietitian through a medical center. I suggest you work with a registered dietitian—someone with an R.D. degree. Stay away from anyone who professes to be a "nutritionist." You often find less-than-qualified nutrition advisers working in health clubs and health food stores, and they typically want you to buy a host of supplements and vitamins.

- **Chest X-ray:** The chest X-ray makes an image of the size of your heart and allows us to look at the presence or absence of spots in your lungs. Some studies suggest that in the nonsmoker who is generally healthy, the chest X-ray is not a consistently helpful tool, but it continues to be ordered.

- **EKG:** This is a tracing of your heart, known as an electrocardiogram. You see these on TV doctor shows all the time. The patient is hooked up to 12 wires, which are attached with sticky pads in an array across your bare chest. It's not a shock or uncomfortable or painful at all. The EKG measures your heart rhythm and prints out a strip of blips. This test is a general screen for any evidence of heart disease. Doctors can tell from the pattern what may be going on if you have irregular heart rhythms or problems.

- **Vision and hearing screening:** Most doctors don't conduct vision exams like you would have done at a vision center where you might be fitted for eyeglasses. But if you have any medical problems with your eyes, your doctor would refer you to a medical doctor called an ophthalmologist for a further check. Hearing screening, too, is best performed by an audiologist in a soundproof room with sophisticated equipment. Structural ear problems can be addressed if you are referred to an ear, nose, and throat specialist.

- **Immunization review and update:** Adults need shots, too, just like children do. The Centers for Disease Control and Prevention (CDC) annually updates a schedule of immunizations for adults. This includes a flu shot every year, especially for those at higher risk, such as the elderly and those with weakened immune systems, and now the flu shot or flu mist is recommended for just about everyone. The pneumonia shot is a wise choice. It's just one injection at any age and a revaccination if you're over 65.

  Talk with your doctor about getting protected against hepatitis A and B and screened for C, especially if you're a baby boomer. People working in medical occupations should be fully immunized.

  Tetanus is a once-every-10-years thing, so don't wait to step on a nail in your yard or to be snared by a stray fish hook to get a booster. And if you're a grandparent, you should consider the combination tetanus/diphtheria/pertussis (Tdap) so you don't put your grandchildren at risk, especially for whooping cough, which is pertussis. Some adults may even benefit from catching up their childhood vaccinations for measles, mumps, and rubella, and now you can get a one-time vaccine to prevent shingles (when the dormant chicken pox returns with a vengeance in later life to cause painful patches of blisters).

  Immunizations are especially important if you travel overseas. The CDC has complete tracking on what shots are needed for certain nasty diseases you'd never be exposed to in the United States, depending on where you're headed. I suggest checking the CDC website well in advance of any overseas travel, especially if you're going someplace exotic. Your doctor may refer you to an infectious disease expert.

- **Treadmill exercise test and cardiovascular health clinic consultation:** We really do get physical and put our patients through a treadmill test when we first see them, and then every five years after that initial visit. We tape electrodes for an EKG, the heart tracing, on the chest and put our patients on a treadmill to begin brisk walking. Usually, fatigue signals the end of the test, or we stop the testing if we see abnormalities on the cardiogram.

- **Vitamin B$_{12}$:** We also measure vitamin B$_{12}$ levels to pinpoint a difficult-to-detect disease called pernicious anemia—a condition that shows up in older people. This is easily treated with vitamin B$_{12}$ injections or an oral form of the medication.

- **Colon:** The gold standard for detection of cancer of the colon remains a colonoscopy. Usually this is started at about age 40 or 50, and then repeated every 5 years or so, based on your risk.

- **Bone density:** The role of assessing for the bone-thinning condition known as osteoporosis remains controversial. Most clinicians would recommend a bone density assessment at about the time of menopause for women, or earlier if there is a strong positive family history of disorders that might be associated with osteoporosis, such as for heavy smokers and women who are relatively inactive. We also test bone density in men.

  The test is a quick X-ray of your hip and spine taken while you lie on an X-ray table with your legs elevated on a foam block. Simple. The quick tests done at health fairs and shopping-center screenings, in which bone density is measured through your wrist, finger, or heel, are just mass screening devices for awareness. If you try one of these tests and are judged to have low bone density, get the full spine and hip screening before you and your doctor make any decisions about treatment.

- **Prostate specific antigen (PSA):** Although discussed in detail earlier, this bears repeating. For men, most medical authorities recommend an early PSA starting at age 50, but in the African-American community—especially if there is a strong family history of cancer of the prostate—the PSA is typically started much earlier, even at age 40. But know that many medical organizations are not recommending routine PSA testing.
- **Mammogram:** Again, although discussed earlier, this also bears repeating. Most medical groups recommend annual mammograms, starting at age 40.
- **Pap smear:** A Pap smear usually is performed every one to three years, but more frequently in women who are sexually active or have multiple sexual partners.
- **Mental health:** Most clinicians do not routinely screen for depression unless there are some clear-cut indications of concern. Patients usually don't come in and announce they are depressed, although we are encouraged by campaigns to raise awareness about this highly treatable condition. But if a patient talks about not sleeping, not eating, gaining a lot of weight, or the joy in life just not being there, we can ask leading questions to get to the heart of the matter.

Obviously, the general medical exam needs to be focused on your specific needs, but this is the battery of testing we follow for our patients. Any test or examination by your doctor needs to be carefully interpreted for you, especially laboratory tests that take a few days for results to come back.

I don't think it's enough for you to receive a postcard in the mail with boxes checked that say "normal." If you're comfortable with that, fine. But I advise you to discuss your test results by phone with the doctor or in person. That way your questions can be answered on the spot. Tell the doctor you expect to hear from him or her by phone. And continue to follow up with the doctor's office until you get an answer.

Also don't be comforted if the doctor's office says, "We'll call you if you have any abnormal results." You could easily slip through the cracks in a poorly designed alert system like that. Don't settle for a no-news-is-good-news plan. You want to hear the news, whatever it is, even if you have to keep calling the office. **Do it.**

Many patients are asking for lab results and consultation reports to be faxed or e-mailed to them, and if you want copies, set this up before you leave the office. That way, you can add these to the medical record file you are building. Or ask the office to mail you a copy. If they require a release form, sign that before you leave as well.

My Prevention Rx

One of the greatest deterrents to and strongest arsenals against disease is having a relationship with a primary health care professional who can provide access to the medical system and can appropriately interpret signs and symptoms. Equally important, a careful physical examination and a thorough medical history may detect an early-stage illness or developing condition when it is potentially curable and probably controllable.

Screening is a mantra embedded into the fabric of the American Cancer Society. The earlier a cancer (or any disease) is detected and treated, the better the prognosis. **I know of no instance in which the outcome of a far-advanced cancer is better than that of an early-stage cancer.** Therefore, individuals and their health care providers should be in a partnership to outline acceptable screening studies to detect cancer in a curable stage.

Use the health partnership you have created with your doctor, nurse-practitioner, or physician assistant. This is the person you can talk to and in whom you trust. But, ultimately, your health is in your hands. No one has a greater stake in your health than you do. We are each on a journey. An overarching theme of life is to have meaning and purpose. Without that, there is no reason to go on. "Give me a reason to live, and I will find a way to live," wrote Holocaust survivor Viktor Frankl in *Man's Search for Meaning*.

We each have the possibilities, gifts, and talents to remake the world in some small way. But we cannot do that without health—the greatest of all blessings. Give a man a fish, and he will no longer go hungry, but teach him how to fish, and he then learns to feed his soul. In a way, I hope you are learning how to fish ... not for trout but for well-being.

7

Your Prevention Prescription

*Each of us can indeed
make the world a little better than it is right now.
But we have to be here to do that.*

The handwriting is on the wall. Lifestyle choices do make a difference in how well we live and how long we live.

Some studies have shown that our lifestyle/behavior choices and options reflect 75 percent of our quality and length of life. Just think about this: Approximately 40 percent of all cancers are due to the choices we make, not to a roll of the genetic dice. In other words, we can prevent the vast majority of medical miseries, including cancer and heart disease, at least in part, by taking charge of our lives, by being proactive, by being an active participant in health care decisions, and by recognizing that the buck stops with us when it comes to such lifestyle choices as eating and drinking, smoking, sleeping, driving, and exposure to the sun.

With age comes wisdom, and I've gathered some of my best thoughts here to offer you some practical, painless advice for quitting, moderating, and improving in all of the lifestyle areas.

Exercise: The Real Fountain of Youth

*The most significant muscles you need
to stay out of a nursing home
are the thigh muscles.*

I can't take out my pad and write a prescription for any medicine more powerful than exercise. Here's why.

When I speak to audiences across the country, I take a gallon of milk with me on stage. Why? Because 70 percent of women and 25 percent of men in the audience will not be able to lift that full gallon of milk—weighing about 10 pounds—by the time they reach age 70. After age 70, many people can't get themselves up off the floor without assistance. Or out of a chair. Just think about that.

After age 30, we truly are over the hill as far as our muscles are concerned. At that point, we start to lose muscle mass and flexibility. Our older folks assume a crouch as they age—much of that is nature's way of creating stability.

The individual who does not have the flexibility to bend forward is at higher risk for falls, which may result in hip fractures and other serious problems. Take note: The most significant muscles you need to stay out of a nursing home are the thigh muscles. As these weaken, older people become unstable, they fall, they buy a one-way ticket to a nursing home, and their golden years quickly tarnish.

As a society, we have obviously become couch potatoes. Most of us don't get off the sofa to change the TV channel—we use the remote. An equal number of us don't even get out of our cars to open the garage door—we use the remote—and rarely do we walk instead of drive. Surprisingly, no one uses a remote to open the refrigerator door, but I suspect that's next.

We have become meat eaters and sedentary, and in some areas of the country, at least 69 percent of people are overweight or obese. Eighty percent of Americans do not meet regular physical activity guidelines. In the 10 years between the first edition of this book and this writing, these numbers have increased steadily. It scares me to think about where we will wind up unless we start to take personal responsibility for our health.

Increasing numbers of our fellow Americans are growing rounder, and obesity is especially tragic among children and adolescents. As we've seen, long-term studies of aging unequivocally demonstrate that a sedentary lifestyle is as much a risk factor for early death as smoking, high cholesterol, and high blood pressure. Studies are clearly showing that sitting is a risk factor.

When it comes to cancer, there is no doubt in my mind that the physically fit fare far better with cancer than those who are unfit. Regular exercise appears to reset certain body systems, such as hormone production and fat stores, that are disrupted if you are overweight or obese.

A new definition of exercise

The real Fountain of Youth is indeed physical activity. But what is meant by physical activity anyway?

Performing yoga sun salutations in morning light. Kayaking as the sun sets on a tranquil lake. Dancing to a favorite song. Strolling through the neighborhood park while holding the hand of your grandchild. Pruning rose bushes. These are the movements of a happy, healthy life. And these are the movements your body craves and needs.

Researchers at Kent State found that people whose exercise regimen consists of tapping their thumbs on their smartphones have lower fitness levels. They even proposed a new name for high users of cell phones: phone potatoes.

The benefits of physical activity in terms of improved self-esteem, positive body image, and a sense of wellness can be spectacular.

For heart-healthy exercise, the American Heart Association advocates a gradual program so that you can comfortably walk and talk for 30 to 60 minutes 5 times a week. How much is that? Just a few hundred minutes of walking (and talking if you have a partner) per week. You probably use more cellphone time than that each week.

The Institute of Medicine recommends at least 60 minutes of moderately intense physical activity each day to prevent weight gain and achieve the full health benefits of activity. In contrast, the U.S. Surgeon General, together with the American College of Sports Medicine and

National Institutes of Health, says health benefits can be obtained from three 10-minute walks a day (total of 30 minutes daily).

The President's Council on Fitness, Sports & Nutrition, in setting the Physical Activity Guidelines for Americans, recommends 30 minutes daily for adults. That's 150 minutes a week of moderate-intensity exercise (10 minutes at a time counts too).

So which is it: 60 minutes or 30? No one knows for sure, and certainly an expert panel can't tell you what is best for you. The answer may be somewhere in between. Experts recommend that sedentary adults try to build up to 60 minutes of moderate intensity per day, which may also reduce the risk of weight gain over time and will provide additional health benefits beyond 30 minutes of activity per day.

Anything to get millions of couch-bound Americans off the cushions and onto their feet is a start. Did you know that walking at a pace of 3.5 miles per hour, a 150-pound person burns about 5 calories every minute? In front of the TV, that same person burns just one calorie per minute. At least stand up during those commercials and move around.

Lasting behavior change comes slowly, so don't throw up your hands at the suggestion that 60 minutes is what you need and then do nothing because the barriers seem overwhelming. Start somewhere: Take the first step, then build up to your comfort zone.

If you're wondering if you're working out too hard or not hard enough, be patriotic and take the talk test. If you can't say the Pledge of Allegiance comfortably, you're working out too hard. The talk test provides a simple and reliable indicator of the proper training intensity for runners, according to the researchers who asked study participants to recite the pledge during harder and harder running speeds.

At some point, a workout becomes too intense, and you simply can't talk (or say the Pledge of Allegiance or sing). That's the point. You want to back off on your intensity.

The Aerobic Mile

An aerobic mile, simply, is how much energy you expend jogging one mile. Okay, you don't want to jog. But you can burn the same number of calories by doing other forms of exercise. Here are some examples of activities you can do to equal one aerobic mile:

- Walking 1 mile at any pace
- Bicycling at a moderate pace for 12 minutes
- Vigorous rowing for 12 minutes
- Swimming for 24 minutes
- Tennis for 20 minutes (11 minutes if your game is vigorous)
- Weight training at a moderate pace for 15 minutes
- Easy gardening for 60 minutes
- Aerobic exercise to music, at an easy pace, for 20 minutes
  Beginning exercisers should strive to achieve the equivalent of 6 aerobic miles a week. Those with good fitness levels can move up to 10 miles a week. High fitness levels are achieved with 15 aerobic miles each week, according to ACSM's *Guidelines for Exercise Testing.*

Use it or lose it

This is not a new mantra. I'm talking about lifting weights. But I'm not referring to the ripple-chested, bronze Hercules of the magazines, nor am I referring to a goddesslike creature with flowing blonde hair and a 24-inch waist. I'm referring to you and me. This is one piece of the physical fitness puzzle that has been dramatically underemphasized.

Many people wince at the thought of lifting weights, but the studies are convincing and user friendly. A good first step is an examination by a medical caregiver to be sure you're physically fit. This seems rather odd because what reason could anyone possibly have for not exercising? But just be sure you don't have some type of heart disease or severe osteoporosis. In which case, I still want you to exercise, but you will need to modify your exercise—go slowly, and you should be fine. Second, if the green light is given, follow some simple rules:

- Seek guidance from a certified personal trainer (lots of people say they are trainers; ask for their credentials) or a physical therapist. Just one visit with a pro can help you determine the weight to start with and the proper technique. You can be your own coach after that.

- Start using hand weights such as barbells (soup cans are the frugal version of barbells and much less expensive; or fill empty plastic milk cartons with water or sand) to determine the weight you can easily lift.

- A reasonable program is determined by how much you can lift with ease. Determine the maximum weight you can comfortably lift, let's say, with one arm. If that's 10 pounds, you would take approximately 80 percent of that (or 8 pounds) as the baseline weight for lifting. Let's suppose a biceps curl can be done with 20 pounds; 80 percent of that is 16 pounds.

- A sensible program consists of 8 to 12 repetitions (called a set), so that the last rep is at the point of maximum muscle fatigue. You're really pushing yourself on that one. Most of the benefit of weight lifting occurs with only one set. To do multiple sets may increase strength but only by a small percentage. The biggest bang for the buck is with one set of 8 to 12 repetitions.

- Lifting weights on an every-other-day basis strengthens muscles and can help avoid osteoporosis and other significant health problems. We are in the era of time crunch, so it would be far better to carefully perform one set so that the last repetition is to the point of maximum exertion, meaning you could not lift the weight even one more time.

- On the "other" days of the week, perform your cardio exercise—walking, water aerobics, jogging, cycling, treadmill, step aerobics, Zumba—something that gets your heart rate up.

Lift weights, lose weight. Makes sense. Miriam E. Nelson, Ph.D., internationally known author and professor of nutrition at Tufts University, created news worldwide when her research results were first published in *JAMA*. After a year of strength training twice a week, women's bodies were 15 to 20 years more youthful.

With exercise and strength training, and without drugs, women in her studies regained bone, thus reversing osteoporosis. They became stronger—in most cases even stronger than when they were younger. Their balance and flexibility improved. They were leaner and trimmer, while eating as much as ever. They were better able to avoid falls. What's more, the women were so energized, they became more active. No other program—whether diet, medication, or aerobic exercise—has achieved comparable results.

Did I mention that these were older women? Grandmothers. Women who may have never exercised, or who had been active when they were younger but didn't have a regular program of activity as they aged.

At the same time, you can boost metabolism and melt away fat. Because muscle is metabolically active and fat is not, when you increase your muscle mass, you're able to burn more calories, even when at rest.

If strength training works for women—and it does—men should take note. It will work for you, too. It's just that women have never thought about weight lifting as part of their exercise regimen—until now.

And what about those ab machines? If you absolutely, positively must work your abdominal muscles separately, you've probably been lured into buying an ab exerciser. If you've been up late at night watching infomercials for expensive equipment guaranteed to tighten up those flabby abdominal muscles, you may have already spent too much time—and money—on stuff that may not work.

The absolute truth came out about the tubular metal devices with names such as Ab Roller and ABSculptor in the *Journal of Strength and Conditioning Research*. Researchers in California tested the machines and found they were no better than regular crunches (some of us know these as sit-ups).

Putting activity back into life

Society, of course, doesn't make exercise easy. "You find very few jobs today that require physical activity," observed Paul Ribisl, Ph.D., chair of the department of health and exercise science at Wake Forest University. "We've been so clever at taking physical activity *out*

159

of our lives." Most Americans sit down at work and move only their mouths and their fingers.

"We were given the gift of time and blew it," said Dr. Ribisl. "We've taken the drudgery out of housework and occupations, but we're too foolish to know the time that was saved should be spent on family, friends, self-enrichment, and exercise. Our machine only works if you exercise it."

It's never too late to exercise. Researchers always suspected that brisk walking would outrun, or at least be comparable to, other exercise, and an eight-year study published in the *New England Journal of Medicine* of thousands of female nurses is strong evidence. Women in the study who became active in middle adulthood or later were able to lower their risk for coronary heart disease just by brisk walking 3 or more hours per week (at a pace of at least 3 miles per hour, or 1 mile in 20 minutes).

So take 30 minutes each day. You'll get the same heart-healthy benefits as those who exercise vigorously, and walking is easy and free. You just need a pair of comfortable shoes and a commitment to yourself.

Oh, you don't have time? Make activity work. When I'm traveling, for example, I walk the airport concourse. Did you know that there is a walking track inside the Dallas/Fort Worth International Airport? The track (7/10 of a mile) is aligned with floor medallions in Terminal D from gates D6 to D40. Add stair climbing instead of the escalators along the route, and you have a ready-made workout.

One of my colleagues at Mayo Clinic helped develop the Trek Desk—a working surface for a desk and computer is perched over a treadmill. The user walks slowly while performing all the activities of a normal office staffer. Some call centers have treadmill desks. Customer service reps sign up to use the treadmill station an hour at a time, and my sources say the employees can't get enough of this activity. There's hope.

Daily tasks are not a chore, unless you can't do them. Opening a jar of pickles, getting up out of a chair, climbing a flight of stairs. They seem like simple daily activities, but if you don't have the muscle strength to do them, you can lose your independence, and your quality of life may never be the same.

My Exercise Rx

When it comes to exercise, you're more likely to do as I say than as I do, but keep in mind I'm years in the making. Generally I'm up and out of bed at 4:30 a.m. on most days of the week for 60 minutes of either high-impact aerobics or a Stairmaster set on interval training at level 10 (the highest workout). On some days, I will simply hit the road for an eight-mile run without the gym, and longer runs on weekends or when training for a marathon. Why? I just need to be alone.

Each of these exercise sessions is preceded by 30 seconds of gentle stretching and followed by 60 seconds of vigorous stretching of each major muscle group. Three days a week, I also lift free weights—one or two sets of about 12 repetitions, with the final rep at maximum fatigue. Or I use resistance bands. On the other weekdays, I run, saving the longer 10-mile runs for the weekend days.

Never do I lift weights for the same muscles on consecutive days. And Thursday is an easy "day of rest." What do I give up for this exercise regimen? I need to be tucked into bed by 9:00 p.m.

I am a marathoner. Growing up as a skinny little kid in New Jersey, I was told that because I had no dates, no social skills, and no athletic talents, I had better become a distance runner. I am fortunate to be orthopedically gifted: I have run 14 marathons and have never been seriously injured. I have been able to run almost every day for over 60 years.

In training for a marathon, it is not a question of wishful thinking. I map out a plan and work out day by day, week by week, month by month, so that when the gun goes off on the starting line and I am looking down the barrel of 26.2 miles, I am physically prepared to go the distance—and mentally ready. I have to visualize my goal and take those small successes one step at a time.

It is impossible to envision running 26.2 miles. But if I see myself running the first 5 miles, the second 5 miles, and so on, I can do it. At mile 20, many of my colleagues hit the wall—a runner's term for thinking you just can't take one more step. But we runners *do* take that painful step. We press on even though we think we can't. And you can too. For me, that 20-mile marker means I have only 6.2 miles to go. That is 10,000 meters or 10K, which is a common distance for road races. I can grind it out because I have done my homework, and I am prepared.

The lesson is that we all must run small races. In doing so, see yourself winning and moving on. Enjoy the journey. Then you'll never hit the wall.

Nutrition:
You Are What You Put in Your Grocery Cart

Everything you need,
you can get from food.

Ladies Home Journal sent a reporter and a photographer to follow my wife, Peggy, and me around the grocery store. The story they eventually printed was rather short. So let me give you the long version—with lots of important information before we get to the store—because, as Peggy reminds me every day, we really are what we put in our grocery carts.

Peggy is a registered dietitian. Patients leave the cardiac-care units and come to see her to manage their heart problems, with diet. They meet with Peggy to discuss the eating habits that may have led to their heart disease. If they didn't know before, they leave armed with the best information available on food content and dietary choices, and a renewed sense of empowerment that they can make positive changes in their diets.

Like all behavior, you need a good reason to change your eating habits. Being a patient in a cardiac unit is one. Surviving a heart attack is another. (One-third of people who have heart attacks don't survive.) And being overweight contributes to heart disease.

There's a distinction between being "overweight" and being "obese." In adults, obesity can be defined as a waist circumference greater than 40 inches for men and greater than 35 inches for women. You don't actually need a tape measure to figure this one out. Just look at the belts hanging in your closet, including the ones that are too small.

One-fourth of the population is currently on a "diet," and another 54 percent makes conscious efforts to achieve weight control, according to a national survey released by the Calorie Control Council, a nonprofit association of manufacturers of low-calorie, reduced-fat, and "light" foods and beverages. This is an interesting group to be talking about diets. Theoretically, so-called light foods should have contributed to shrinking Americans instead of widening them. But "reduced-fat," "fewer calories," and "light" gave eaters a false promise of easy weight control. Low-fat cookies still contain calories, and therein lies the problem.

Simple Math

A calorie is the amount of energy stored in food. When you eat more calories than your body can use, you store that extra energy, mostly as fat, and then you gain weight.

I'm not laying blame for an epidemic of obesity in America, but when I wrote the original version of this book 10 years ago, Yankee Stadium had yanked out its seats and replaced them with fewer yet wider seats to accommodate its growing fans. Now it's common to see wider everything, from chairs and bus seats, to wider bathroom stalls and stairways. Airlines and auto makers have seat belt extenders. Hospitals are accommodating supersized patients with wider wheelchairs, bigger gurneys and blood pressure cuffs, and specialized surgical tools, needles, and tubes. Even coffins have been made larger.

Perhaps it's time we concentrate less on "diet" and "dieting" and more on permanent behavior change habits regarding healthy eating. Successful weight management will follow. Over the long haul, "diets" do not work.

We've all seen (and maybe tried) the popular quick-fix diets. But what is their logical conclusion? That you starve yourself, feel deprived, and continue to drop weight, until you weigh nothing? Maintaining an ideal body weight (ideal for you, not for a fashion model or movie star) means a lifelong commitment to healthful eating and exercise, not an on-again, off-again scheme.

At Mayo Clinic, we are often asked about the Mayo Clinic Diet. It was an Internet hoax, an urban legend. These "miracle" diets have been circulating erroneously and had nothing to do with our clinic, by the way. When asked about them, we would say, "There's no such thing." What we offer is a sound, individualized eating plan for life.

In 2010, however, my colleagues developed and published *The Mayo Clinic Diet: Eat Well, Enjoy Life, Lose Weight,* which spells out a doable and successful program that I completely agree with.

Calories count

Calories *do* count for most people, and what is crucial is caloric density, which is the number of calories packed into a measured volume of food. A tiny little Halloween-sized candy bar packs a huge caloric punch and won't fill you up; whereas, you may not be able to finish a bowl of less-calorie-dense air-popped popcorn. Which would be a better snack choice?

Feeling full depends on eating a satisfying amount of food. Eat a large bowl of grapes instead of a handful of raisins (same number of calories). One will fill you up while the other will leave you foraging in your refrigerator for more food.

A note about water: You still need your six to eight 8-ounce glasses per day. I suggest you make water your beverage of choice with every meal and between them.

Fad diets can be as tantalizing as the forbidden foods they promise you can eat while losing weight. The currently popular diets work, and you will lose weight—but for all the wrong reasons.

Basic truth # 1: You can't follow a fad diet forever. You lose weight on popular high-protein diets, for example, because you're cutting out carbohydrates (potatoes and pasta, breads, fruits and vegetables) that usually make up at least half of your daily calorie intake. But it's not the switch to more protein or busting a "sugar" habit blamed on carbohydrates that causes you to lose weight. It's the decrease in carbohydrates that causes the weight loss.

The diet doctors who write bestselling books don't tell you it's almost impossible to stay on a high-protein, low-carbohydrate diet.

The reality is that you can't eat steak and bacon every day or drink the liquid-protein diet drinks that celebrities promote for the rest of your life, nor should you try. When the diet stops, your weight returns with a vengeance because your body quickly replaces lost muscle and fat. I see this played out with patients almost every day.

Basic truth #2: On a diet, your body is starving. Eating a lot of protein alone is dangerous and may eventually lead to a condition called ketosis, in which your body creates toxic levels of ketones that may damage your kidneys beyond repair. Besides causing bad breath and nausea, the ketone production drastically changes your metabolism. You create a condition (much like in famine-stricken people) in which your body will do just the opposite of what you want—instead of processing food normally, everything you eat will fatten you up.

Here's the trap: High-protein diets often equate to taking in too much saturated fat in meats, which may raise cholesterol levels, thus posing an even higher risk for heart problems.

At the other end of the dieting spectrum, just fruit-and-vegetable diets that are extremely low in fat can be dangerous because they often don't supply needed calcium, protein, and other nutrients. Besides, vegetarian-type diets may not appeal to everyone. Those trying to keep fat intake below 10 or 20 percent often don't feel satisfied without animal protein and eventually must add lean cuts of meat and fish to fill the nutritional gap. The bottom line is this: Any diet that excludes certain foods may not be helpful.

The take-home lesson is that we usually want to eat the same volume of food (that's why restrictive diets don't work). Best strategy: Select high-volume foods bulked up with vegetables, for example, and then eat as much food as you normally do. You'll take in fewer calories yet feel satisfied and "full." So much for cheesecake snack bars. Besides, could one possibly be enough?

A key finding: Research on successful dieters—those who have kept weight off for years—shows that they limit the number of fat calories by paying attention to nutrient density. In other words, they know the advantages of an apple over a candy bar. They have strong social support systems, which I know keeps you well. And, just as important, they have incorporated a physical activity program into their lives. You knew I'd work the exercise part in somewhere.

Above all, psychologists say, behavior determines our health. Just knowing what to do doesn't mean you'll do it. Again, it's the old "I know I should lose weight but …" rationalization. Successful dieters must actually make behavior changes to add exercise to their lives.

How much should you weigh?

Another commonly asked question is this: *How much should I weigh?* The rule of thumb for men is 106 pounds for the first 60 inches of height; then 6 pounds per inch over the first 60 inches. So a reasonable weight for a man at 5 feet, 9 inches in height would be 106 + (9 x 6 inches), or 160 pounds. For women, use 105 pounds for the first 60 inches and 5 pounds per inch after that. These are just general guidelines.

Maintaining a trim weight, ideal for your height and build, can be done. Let me put in a convincing plug for having more plant-based meals. The evidence from the research labs is compelling.

Plant-based foods are rich in vitamins, minerals, fiber, and beneficial substances called phytochemicals (*phyto* means "plant"). All may protect against some cancers. In addition, plant-based foods are generally low in fat and calories. They have the added bonus of helping you maintain a healthy weight.

If a food comes from a plant, eat it often. Fruits, vegetables, legumes, roots, tubers, 100% whole grains, and whole-grain products, such as wheat bread and cereals, should make up the bulk of your diet. They are high in fiber and have a low amount of fats, which are factors in heart disease and possibly for some cancers, such as breast, colon, and prostate. Legumes include beans (such as black beans, pinto beans, and chickpeas), split peas, and lentils. Common roots and tubers are turnips, beets, potatoes, and sweet potatoes.

Some colleagues found that quercetin—a plant-based nutrient found most abundantly in apples, onions, tea, and red wine—may provide a new method for impacting prostate cancer. Because this cancer usually causes no symptoms, we often don't catch it until it reaches an advanced stage. In a laboratory study, quercetin reduced or prevented the growth of human prostate cancer cells by blocking activity of androgen (male) hormones. Previous research has linked androgens to prostate cancer's development and progression.

Although these results are still early, quercetin may be a potential nonhormonal approach to preventing or treating prostate cancer. This could lend even further credence to the adage about an apple a day.

Or how about a handful of black raspberries a day? Here's another potentially powerful biological weapon for your health. A mix of compounds hiding deep inside the juicy sweetness of black raspberries seemed to hold off tumor formation and progression in rats. Although we'd have to eat several bowls of black raspberries each day to get as much as the rats were fed, it's still sound advice to get your five servings (or more) a day of fruits and vegetables.

Strawberries and blueberries also have chemopreventive agents in them, such as anthocyanins, phenols, and vitamins A, C, E, and folic acid. So make one of your daily servings berries.

Fruit also contains fiber that has another job. As Dr. Robert Lustig says in his book *Fat Chance: The Bitter Truth about Sugar,* squeeze six oranges and drink the juice. You'll get a ton of sugar. But try to peel and eat those six oranges, and you'll be ready to stop well before orange number 5. It's the body's built-in fiber regulator that can control sugar intake, and most of us never get enough fiber.

If you must have food that comes from an animal or is a snack, choose the low-fat version. To cut your fat intake, use low-fat dairy products, choose lean cuts of meat, and use vegetable oils. Generally, poultry, such as whitemeat chicken and turkey, are lower in fat than red meats, such as beef, lamb, and pork (which contrary to their marketing is not the "other" white meat). Loin cuts of red meats can be low in fat if chosen carefully.

Raw nuts are also an excellent snack in limited amounts (a small handful, about a quarter cup).

If you must snack, pick items low in fat and choose baked snacks over fried any day.

Let's talk about biochemistry. Some evidence shows that, as we age, chemicals called free radicals are produced by the body. These chemicals in some circumstances can stir things up. They may be able to ignite or start the growth of cancer. These chemicals are thought to possibly have a connection with the development of heart disease too.

If we can block the development of these free radicals by taking nutritional supplements called antioxidants, there is the hope that the cancer may not occur or that the heart disease might not develop. We're not exactly sure how such antioxidants as vitamin C and vitamin E work, but they may have something to do with slowing both the development of cancer and the aging process.

The Secret of Longevity (Isn't So Secret)

My collaborator had the great fortune to interview one of the world's premier researchers on longevity. He is Professor Emeritus, Dr. Denham Harman. He is perhaps the best example of his research into what makes humans live and what makes them die. He's 98 years old at this writing.

"I'm still around," he said. His crushing handshake is testament to years of tennis (that's one secret to longevity: exercise).

As a young man, Dr. Harman worked in the chemistry labs of Shell Oil in California for almost 15 years. He still holds 35 U.S. patents on such scientific advances as extreme pressure additives and compounds that make fly strips so effective.

Along his career path, he said, "I had the good fortune to work with famous people." Those included Ernest Lawrence, inventor of the cyclotron, and Robert Oppenheimer, father of the atomic bomb. He shrugs it off as "just plain luck."

In the course of his studies, he completed a doctorate in chemistry at the University of California–Berkeley, and later earned an M.D. in internal medicine at Stanford, which quenched his interest in the biology of human life.

"There was a whole field of knowledge we knew nothing about, so at age 33, I went to medical school," he said (second secret: be a lifelong learner; third secret: pursue your passion).

While treating cancer patients at the famous Donner Laboratory in Berkeley, his academic and career preparation led him to ask, "Everything dies. Why?" The scientist in him wanted to figure it out.

A little-known article entitled "Tomorrow You May Be Younger" appeared in a 1945 issue of *Ladies Home Journal.* The article summarized the work of an obscure Russian scientist and piqued Dr. Harman's interest in answering the question about why we die.

"I felt there had to be some common basic cause that killed everything," he told colleagues via videotape sent to a scientific meeting in Portugal entitled "Free Radical Theory of Aging—50 Years and Beyond."

The scientific world was celebrating Dr. Harmon's theory: Free radicals—those highly reactive molecules in the body that are freed in the normal chemical processes of living—cause aging and cell death. That's as detailed as this book will get about the science part.

Dr. Harman pursued his curiosity on the campus of the University of Nebraska Medical Center, where he went in 1958 to prove his theory.

"Mother Nature is very bright," he said. "In the human race, we know the maximum life span is about 85 years. The main objective is to try to increase our functional life span." In other words, live your life as fully as you can.

"Today we can say aging itself is due to the free radicals, which we produce ourselves, plus free radicals which are hitting us from everywhere else, including ionized radiation from the air," he said.

And his once-skeptical colleagues now agree. Dr. Harman is recognized as the father of the free radical theory of aging.

He was nominated for a Nobel Prize in Medicine in 1995, based on his theory.

His work in Nebraska laid the groundwork for continuing research the world over in the aging process and in the discovery of the potential of antioxidants to fight off the damage from free radicals that can cause cancer, heart disease, and other effects of aging.

In the event that he has the inside track on aging, Dr. Harman shared his remaining secrets to longevity. He takes an alphabet soup of antioxidant vitamins to counteract the effects of those free radicals he has been chasing all his life in the laboratory.

Vitamins, such as C, D, E, and CoQ10, are readily available at any drugstore. However, the benefit of these supplements is unclear. Eat fresh, not processed fruits and vegetables, he said. Be active, whether it's yard work, walking, or playing tennis. And challenge your mind every day. He reads journals and novels.

Despite all the advances in medicine, despite better food and housing, Dr. Harman said, "Average life expectancy has reached a plateau. There is an inborn aging process."

"Accept the fact that you're not going to live forever," he said.

Can we prolong life? "No," he said, "but if you work at it, you might make 100." He's nearly there.

A tremendous gap exists between the research in the laboratory and the practical application of this research in your life. In general, antioxidants obtained from dietary sources (what you eat) are probably better than the antioxidants you buy in a tablet form at Walgreens. At one time, some researchers suggested that vitamin E, for example, would be helpful against heart disease, but that issue has not been proven. Likewise, the role of antioxidants as a way to prevent cancer, while theoretically appealing, has not withstood the scrutiny of rigorously conducted clinical trials.

Low-fat dairy foods, such as milk, yogurt, and cheese, may help control body fat. Here's how: Mistakenly, people may cut out milk, yogurt, and cheese when trying to control or lose weight. In actuality, low-fat versions of these dairy foods may help control body fat in a well-balanced daily diet. These low-fat foods also may help reduce your risk for developing osteoporosis—a softening of bones that may lead to breaks—because they contain the calcium needed to keep bones strong.

Most men don't realize they're at risk for osteoporosis too. It's no longer a condition reserved just for older women. Drinking milk and doing weight-bearing exercise can greatly increase men's chances of keeping bones strong now and later in life. Like women, men ages 19 to 50 need at least three 8-ounce glasses of milk or calcium-fortified food, such as orange juice, each day to help meet the recommended 1,000 milligrams of calcium (women over 51 should strive for 1,200 milligrams). Government data confirm that 7 out of 10 men are not meeting these recommendations.

Vitamin D—What You Need to Know

Without vitamin D, your bones may not grow strong at any age. Why? Because for your bones to make the best use of calcium, they need vitamin D, we are told by Dr. Robert P. Heaney, researcher and professor in the Osteoporosis Research Center at Creighton University.

But did you know that even mild shortages of vitamin D can contribute to diabetes, some cancers, high blood pressure, heart disease, and pregnancy problems?

"Asking the body to deal with these disorders without adequate vitamin D is like asking a fighter to enter battle with one hand tied behind his back," said Dr. Heaney.

Vitamin D is a chemical that our body's tissues use to produce biochemical products required for daily life. It's less important to understand the process. It's more important to know where to get vitamin D and how much you need.

Some facts:

- Your skin produces vitamin D when you are exposed to certain rays of the sun. If you never get sunshine on your skin, you will not get enough ultraviolet radiation for your skin to make vitamin D. This is a tricky balance between getting some sunshine to make vitamin D and reducing your risk for skin cancer from the sun's ultraviolet rays.
- Sunlight in winter in most of the U.S. (and certainly where I live in the North country) is so weak, it does not allow you to produce enough vitamin D, even if you're outside in winter during midday.
- During summer months, a light-skinned person wearing a bathing suit will make about 15,000 IU (international unit) of vitamin D in 15 to 20 minutes. Darker-skinned people can do the same, but it will take twice as long.
- Sunscreen blocks the radiation and prevents your skin from making vitamin D. Brief sun exposure, said Dr. Heaney, is not enough to cause skin cancer. He suggested you apply sunscreen after the first 15 minutes in the sun.
- Some food has vitamin D but not much. Vitamin D is added to many foods, such as fortified milk, fish, eggs, and some yogurt and orange juice, cheese, and breakfast cereals. Read the labels to see how much vitamin D is in the product.
- Because most of us do not get enough sun exposure (or choose not to) or enough vitamin D in food, Dr. Heaney suggests taking supplements of vitamin D_3, the natural form. The label should say cholecalciferol (vitamin D_3); or ask the pharmacist which supplement is best.
- Vitamin D is safe to take.
- You may take supplements daily, weekly, or monthly. The important point is that you need to maintain a high enough blood level of vitamin D. This is measured by a blood test.

- Dr. Heaney recommends, based on his research, that the body needs at least 4,000 IU per day to meet that blood level. But not all experts agree on the dose. Always check with your health care provider. Even sun and food can provide no more than 2,000 IU per day. He says adults should take supplements providing from 1,000 to 3,000 IU per day. This number is higher than the Institute of Medicine recommends. But Dr. Heaney said the officially recommended intakes are a minimum level.
- Talk with your doctor about testing your blood level, and discuss how much supplementation you may need in both summer and winter.

Obesity is a known risk factor for several major types of cancer. Cancers of the breast, the gallbladder, the uterus, and the kidney seem to occur in excess among individuals who are over their ideal body weight.

As with all cancers, colon cancer is an example where early detection virtually assures cure and a final victory. Although there is ongoing controversy, by increasing the fiber and decreasing the fat in our diet (and adding physical activity), we can increase our odds of avoiding this problem in the first place. Still, early detection and screening are absolutely vital.

Cancer of the uterus, although an infrequent cause of cancer death among women, also seems to be related to obesity and dietary issues. Firm data and solid numbers are elusive, but the drift of evidence suggests that women who can maintain an ideal body weight may well decrease their risk of that cancer as well.

You can "fiberize" your kitchen. Stock up with whole grains and fiber-containing foods from cupboard to refrigerator to freezer, according to Anita Kobuszewski, R.D., author of *Food: Field to Fork, How to Grow Sustainably, Shop Wisely, Cook Nutritiously, and Eat Deliciously*. She tells us, "Remember—nutrition doesn't begin until the food passes your lips."

Life in the fast-food lane

The *Reader's Digest* version of an adequate daily eating guide is this: Multiply your weight in pounds times 10. Therefore, at 180 pounds, you would require approximately 1,800 calories per day. A sedentary person may feel comfortable with this number; conversely, a laborer may require more calories, but at least it's a starting point.

A general guideline would divide these 1,800 calories as follows:

- 15 to 20 percent protein
- 55 to 60 percent carbohydrates
- 25 to 30 percent fat

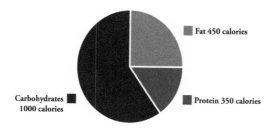

Fat 450 calories

Carbohydrates 1000 calories

Protein 350 calories

Pay special attention to the fats because saturated fats, such as butter and lard, are factors in coronary artery disease, along with trans fats found mainly in partially hydrogenated foods (avoid any fats that are solid at room temperature). Best choices for fats are monounsaturated fats, such as olive, canola, and peanut oils. Because there are 9 calories per gram of fat, 450 calories / 9 = 50 grams of fat as the maximum for our 180-pound person. It's best to keep fats at less than 60 grams per day. All this information is on food labels.

If you've ever reached for a food item in the grocery store, turned it over, and read the label, chances are you were surprised to see that it was high in fat. Perhaps you simply put it back. Perhaps you held two different brands side by side to compare their labels. The standardization in food labeling makes this type of comparison much easier. After over a decade of such mandatory food labeling, consumers are smarter about high-fat foods on grocery shelves.

Are you always on the go? Too often, dinner is a grab-and-dash(board) affair. Eating healthfully in the fast-food lane can be done. It's all part of that balance between calories and fat and protein, and it all depends, of course, on what else you've eaten that day. Although these foods don't come with easy-to-consult food labels, you can find out what's in them. Most fast-food chains publish their menu contents and break down the nutritional information. Ask for a brochure next time you drive through or check out nutritional information online.

So can you eat healthfully in the fast-food lane? Yes, carefully. Follow these rules:

- Supersized is out. Order individually. Super meals are only super deals if you want high calories and fat content. Order and eat the single burger; toss the bun.
- Get low-fat milk or water instead of a soft drink. No sweetened anything.
- Fruit. Yes, you can get fruit in some fast-food places.
- The salad is usually a better choice. But select your dressing carefully or use only part of the dressing. Dip your fork in the dressing on the side, then stab your lettuce.
- Eat prudently the rest of the day.

Dining out poses its own challenges when you've got the menu propped in front of you. Everything sounds great, and you're about to make a decision based on your level of hunger, which is probably high because that's why you're sitting in a restaurant. Many restaurants these days like to win you over with huge quantities. If you see patrons walking away with white Styrofoam to-go boxes, you can guess the portion size is rather large.

Your best bet is to stick to baked or grilled or broiled items, not fried. Order sauce on the side, or season your pasta or fish or salad with fresh lemon. Salad dressing should be ordered on the side, not dumped on the salad. Instead of butter and sour cream on that baked potato, try salsa or low-fat cottage cheese.

Upscale restaurants may allow you to share an entree and simply charge you for "another plate." It's worth the money, and you won't go away hungry. Or ask your server to put half of your meal in a "doggy bag" (who are we kidding, the dog never sees this stuff) in the kitchen before serving you. What you don't see, you won't miss, and then you'll have a nice white box to take home for tomorrow. It's also quite acceptable to ask for a smaller portion. I can't imagine a restaurant that wouldn't accommodate this request.

Supermarket savvy*

Make a list, check it twice. Before you even walk inside the supermarket, always make a list. If you don't, you will buy stuff you never dreamed you'd have in your cart. At the same time, never go shopping when you're hungry because you'll sample and buy food you had no intention of eating. Don't be tempted to pick up food samples at grocery store demos.

First, sit down and plan out a week's worth of menus. This gets easier the more you do it. Focus on what to have for the main item of the meal. For example, Monday will be chicken, then decide what goes with that. Salad and baked potatoes. Tuesday will be fish. Wednesday is a meatless day. Thursday is hamburgers. Fish again on Friday; and Saturday, roast pork. Then work on what you want to add to those meals.

Change your thinking a little by making meat (protein) the accompaniment to the meal. Make no more than 3 to 4 ounces of meat per person, if you choose to serve meat, which we don't. That's about the size of a deck of cards or a hockey puck, and it's a good "deal." An ideal meal would be a boneless, skinless chicken breast; a small salad with green leafy lettuce and tomatoes, carrots, and cucumber; a cup of steamed broccoli; and a small-to-medium-sized baked potato (about the size of a tennis ball).

Let's talk about salad dressing. A lot of people don't like the taste of the low-fat dressings. Make your own with olive oil and vinegar and a little blue cheese. But, as with fast-food salads, here's the best technique. Put the dressing on the side and dip your fork in the dressing first, then stab the vegetables. It's amazing how much less you'll use. So when you order out, whether fast food or fine dining, request your dressings and sauces on the side, and then use

*This section was developed in consultation with Peggy Menzel, R.D., L.D.

this technique. That way, you have total control over what you put on your food and in your mouth.

For dessert, how about a nice bowl of fresh cut fruit salad, nothing on it? Or spoon some low-fat or nonfat vanilla yogurt over the fruit; leave it drizzled or mix it all together. Greek yogurt, which has taken over the yogurt market, is higher in protein and lower in carbs, and so is recommended for those managing diabetes and for the rest of us. See if you like it.

Take note of the ingredients on the label. If you see *carmine*, you may wish to pass. Carmine is added color made from the crushed bodies of a certain type of beetle. Yes, bugs. It's perfectly okay with the FDA, but it sounds creepy to me.

Cooking is becoming a lost art. No one wants to do much cooking, which is why we turn to convenience foods and fast foods. They're quick and sometimes acceptable for an occasional meal. Try not to get into the habit of making a stop at KFC part of your standard fare. Use a crock pot and make (and freeze) meals ahead. You can make better soup than Campbell's and a better dinner than Swanson. Plan menus and shop accordingly.

However, the roasted chickens so many grocery stores now offer in the delis can brighten up any plate. But take the skin off. Pick the meat off the bones, and make chicken salad the next day.

Shop the perimeter. As your menus come together, your list of ingredients will be building. You'll find that most of the better choices are found around the perimeter of the store. The fresh fruits and vegetables, bakery, meats, frozen foods and dairy are usually arranged around the outside, while the more processed foods are in the center aisles. Your plan is to shop the perimeter and venture into the center only as needed. It's a jungle in there!

If you're like most American shoppers, you'll spend an average of 43 minutes shopping. That's down from 45 minutes in the annual American Time Use Survey conducted by the Bureau of Labor Statistics.

Fruits and vegetables: Spend the majority of your 43 minutes among the fruits and vegetables. Pick out ripe or ripening produce. Your selection will depend on the season, of course, and where you live. In summer, you'll find more melons and better grapes and mangoes. Go for pigment. Choose as many different brilliantly colored fruits as you can, such as strawberries, blueberries, bananas, oranges, apples, and melons.

Your best choices among the vegetables are dark green leafy ones (such as romaine, red leaf lettuce, or spinach—not iceberg lettuce). Select the colorful pigments of carrots, broccoli, peppers (green, red, and orange), green beans, asparagus, and more. When forced to choose, buy less ripe rather than too ripe.

Why go for color? All these foods contain phytochemicals (the good stuff from plants), antioxidants, and fiber.

The Surprising Truth about Organic Foods

Is organic better? *Organic* simply means the fruits and vegetables were grown without pesticides. This may be important to you if you eat the peel on fruits (such as apples). And certainly it's hard to avoid eating the peel on grapes.

When we get home from the store, first, I wash my own hands. Then I wash, rinse, and dry my fruits and veggies to remove any residue. Water works just as well as any special sprays. The important thing is to dry the fruit. Then water won't sit in the bottom of the bowl and cause the produce to go bad. I let everything ripen on the kitchen counter. Some items, such as avocados and pears, do well ripening in a brown-paper bag.

Keep fruit in a pretty bowl or basket on the counter so you'll see (and eat) it.

Peggy prefers mostly organic and likes the taste better. She's a big fan of farmers' markets.

Meat: Continuing around the perimeter of your grocery store, you'll get to the meat section. Some of us choose not to eat meat for various reasons. This is an individual decision. But if you choose to eat meat, some tips will help you use the meat counter to your advantage.

Think small. Think about eating red meat only one or two times a week. The Mediterranean food guide pyramid, based on the heart-healthy diet of our friends in the Greek Islands, puts meat almost in the same category as sweets—limited amounts, not every day. Instead of beef or pork, try fish, poultry, or go meatless. When you choose to have meat, I encourage you to limit portion size to a deck of cards (a single deck!). Women can be guided by the rule of thumb of no more than 5 ounces per day; men about 6 ounces. That deck of cards is about 3 ounces.

So you can see that a pound of ground beef, with the lowest possible fat content, at 16 ounces will go a long way. If you choose not to buy the 95 percent lean burger, buy the higher-fat-content meat, cook it, and then drain it well in a colander, and even rinse it with water to remove fat. The flavor will depend on the seasonings you put into it.

Use ground turkey in place of ground beef, but check your labels; you want ground white turkey meat, not the dark meat or the skin.

You may have heard about and even tried TVP. That's texturized vegetable protein, better known by any other name: soy protein (plant-based). These meat substitutes are virtually indistinguishable from meat if you use them in chili or lasagna, but it may take getting used to if you dress it up with a bun as a hamburger substitute.

When you select meats, go for cuts with the word *loin* in them. These are lean cuts, contain less saturated fat (the bad stuff), and the butchers have probably trimmed off all visible fat. If they haven't, you can.

Chicken is amazingly versatile. A 3-pound package of boneless, skinless breasts can feed a family of four for multiple meals. But take the skin off any chicken you buy before you cook it. If you insist, cook with the skin on to keep the chicken more moist, but take the skin off before you eat it—don't eat the skin.

Dairy: Rounding the corner to the dairy aisle, still along the perimeter of the grocery store, you'll want to pick up skim milk. Actually, 1 percent milk is fine too. Try dairy substitutes such as soy, rice, and almond milk that are fortified with calcium and vitamin D.

Watch the labels on yogurt to make sure you get the low-fat or fat-free varieties with low sugar content. Eating regular yogurt is like eating a dish of ice cream. As I said, Greek yogurt gives you more protein and less carbohydrate, which is especially important for people with diabetes. Low-fat or fat-free yogurt acts like a dessert without the guilt. Add your own fruit. Try it on top of angel food cake or mix it with your breakfast cereal. Also, different brands have different tastes. If you don't like the store brand or a name brand, try another brand.

Add to that apple a day, a glass of milk a day. Milk drinkers scored better on memory and brain function tests, according to a study in the *International Dairy Journal*.

Grains: You may have to venture inside the aisles to get to the bread. Look for a brand with 5 grams of fiber per slice (that's a lot, and that's what bread is for). Compare that with the fiber content for regular "store-bought" breads (1/2 to 2 grams per slice). You'll get 10 grams, of course, with a sandwich, which is more fiber than most people get in a day, but we need it. In fact, we need 25 to 35 grams of fiber every day.

The most important ingredient listed on the label is the flour itself. You want "100 percent whole-wheat flour" listed as the first ingredient on the label. If it's not, put the loaf back and keep reading labels until you find those four magic words. Breads calling themselves *wheat bread* or *whole-wheat* or *whole grain* or *7-* or *12-grain* may not be the real deal. In fact, they may just be the equivalent of plain white bread that's brown. The label tells the whole truth and nothing but. If it's white, do not bite.

Maybe you don't like wheat bread, or your family refuses to eat it. Try a sandwich with one slice of whole-wheat and one slice of white. But if you lose this battle, just make sure whatever you put between the slices is healthy stuff.

Deli: Can you make it past the deli without stopping for the free samples? Actually, the deli case may have some good choices, such as lean cuts of turkey and roast beef. Stay away from processed meats, such as salami or bologna. Avoid the fried chicken, but the roast chicken is usually delicious (without the skin).

Add some cheeses to your meats. Select cheese made with part skim milk, such as mozzarella.

Fresh deli salads are tempting, but avoid those made with mayonnaise bases, such as the potato and macaroni salads. And the marshmallow whipped-cream salads are also to be avoided. If you have the deli make you a sandwich, opt for mustard not mayo, or select light mayo or a tablespoon of hummus.

The Smart Shopper's Guide to Living with Diabetes

You may be among the 19 million Americans who have been diagnosed with diabetes. Or maybe you're one of the 7 million who don't know they have it yet. Here's an even scarier number: 79 million Americans are in a condition called prediabetes.

By 2050, one in three Americans will have diabetes, according to the CDC. And even if you don't have diabetes and aren't at risk, you might live with someone who needs to control blood glucose levels or is at risk. And that means you all need to make sure the right foods find their way into your grocery cart.

The secret to grocery shopping if you have diabetes (or not) isn't a mystery. No foods have to be off limits, but the key, dietitians tell us, is portion size and what else you eat with a meal.

Everything you need to know is right on the food label. You can compare similar foods by checking nutrition labels. The most important items to look for are serving size, total carbohydrates, and fiber, especially if you're managing diabetes. Fiber is your friend.

Quite simply, carbs turn into glucose in the body (some people call this blood sugar or blood glucose). People with diabetes need to pay attention to the amount of carbohydrates they eat, because their bodies just can't process it into energy as well or as quickly as can people without diabetes.

If you've been diagnosed with diabetes, you'll want to know how many carbs you should be limited to at each meal. For some people, it might be 45 to 60 grams at each meal, and 15 to 30 grams for snacks each day. To find out what is best for you, be sure to talk to your doctor, a certified diabetes educator, or a registered dietitian, for an individualized eating plan.

Here are some tips:

- Spend time in the fruits and veggies aisle, but limit peas, corn, potatoes, and beans, which are considered starchy vegetables. Just a half cup of these is recommended if you choose them. Best choices are nonstarchy vegetables, such as leafy greens, broccoli, carrots, peppers, and the like. Choose fresh veggies if available, then frozen, and no-salt-added canned if you must.

- Canned fruits or snack sizes should be in light syrup or "own juice" or water or labeled as "no sugar added." Avoid heavy syrup. Canned sliced peaches, for example, in heavy syrup have 22 grams of carbs, compared to 12 grams in the lite variety. Most dried fruits have sugar, except apricots, peaches, and apples, but just a quarter cup (2 oz.) is all it takes to add up to 24 grams of carbs. Your best choice is that fresh peach with just 12 grams of carbs.

- Use the serving size on the label to judge which breakfast cereal to buy. Fiber One Honey Squares, for example, says three-quarters of a cup (6 oz.) has 25 grams of carbs. But because it also contains 10 grams of fiber (and you can deduct half the fiber over 5 grams according to the American Diabetes Association), the actual carb count would be 20 grams. Compare that to Special K Protein Plus. The same size serving has 19 grams of carbs and only 3 grams of fiber. The 10 grams of protein, however, will make you feel full longer. Either is a smart choice.

- Bypass the soft drinks, and select an unsweetened iced tea. Add a lemon wedge. Water is still the absolute best drink.

- Snack time offers a multitude of smart choices. A Larabar, for example, is a snack bar with three simple ingredients. Avoid high-calorie protein bars, which can be as fat- and calorie-filled as a Snickers. Or stock up on the 100-calorie packs of everything from mini-cookies to cheese crackers, yogurt-covered pretzels, or brownies. At just 15 grams of carbs, most of these are nicely portable for that desk drawer at work, purse, gym bag, or car.

- A handful of almonds or walnuts may be higher in fat, but they can be a smart snack choice. If that pitiful little handful of nuts doesn't make you think you're eating enough, try popcorn. The microwave mini-bags pop up about 3 cups, and you can eat it all without guilt.

- Deli meat with a slice of cheese can be sandwiched between two slices of 100 percent whole-wheat or whole-grain bread, as long as those words are the first ingredient listed on the bread label. Pepperidge Farm Light Style Soft Wheat offers two slices at 16 grams of total carbs. Sara Lee Delightful is another fine choice with 19 grams of carbs and 5 grams of fiber.

- Add a Greek yogurt to a meal. Why Greek? Because this style boosts the protein and lowers the carbs in the way the product is produced. Liquid is strained away, and along with that goes a lot of the carbohydrate.

- When it comes to meat, think about playing cards. That's the portion size (3 ounces) of chicken, fish, or red meat. Prepare your meat by baking, grilling, or roasting.

- For an occasional special treat, dessert can be a piece of cake 2 inches square or a homemade cookie.

Is one-a-day enough or even necessary?

Now let me say that I'm not opposed to vitamins, but you don't need to overdo it. Everything you need, you can get from food. But a once-a-day multivitamin for added assurance is usually fine for most people. Your doctor may suggest particular supplements for you. But it's my experience that some people who take vitamins often have no idea why or how much they should take, or what the supplements are supposed to be doing.

People who eat a generally healthy diet do not need a multivitamin.

My Nutrition Rx

We really do become what we eat. For me, I do all I can to shift the odds in my favor. In fact, I won't let the airlines dictate what they can serve me. I order a plant-based meal when I make my flight reservations, or I bring my own meal along with healthier snacks. I speak up at restaurants. Of course, I'm not naïve. And I do not believe for a moment that I can avoid cancer or heart disease altogether, but I do believe that I can have a better hand to play if I stay in charge. So can you.

Only you are responsible for what you're putting into your mouth. Because there is no question that excess body weight is responsible for heart disease and some cancers, you can use the tips here to eat defensively for your good health.

From Burnout to Balance

*Phone calls, e-mail, and texts
can quickly become enormous time-wasters
and block your coronary arteries.*

It used to be, if you worked hard, showed up and did your job, your employer would take care of you. That was then. Working Americans now feel disposable and replaceable. And those entering the workforce today can anticipate a minimum of five career shifts in their professional lifetimes—maybe more. And no gold watch at the retirement party.

We counsel high school and college students about portable skills and marketable traits as they put together their portfolios of values and interests. These will be the tools that serve them in their quest and will be there when they need to bounce back as they go from job to job in today's marketplace.

Job security? Gone. Mergers, acquisitions, consolidations, restructuring, and downsizing have created a new Willy Loman, the tragic hero in *Death of a Salesman*—it's all *About Schmidt* and Jack Nicholson's dead-on portrayal in Alexander Payne's brilliant film of what may lie ahead for many Americans when released from the corporate cocoon. We witness the death of these salesmen and saleswomen over and over again.

Long-term employment is a phenomenon of the past. It is unlikely that anyone will spend an entire career under one corporate umbrella anymore, or even under any corporate umbrella. The growth of small business and work-from-home, or at least telecommuting via Internet, is replacing the office cubicle farm. Many corporate umbrellas are imploding under their own ineptitude, dumping disenfranchised employees and disgruntled stockholders. And regardless of your career status, the skills required to maintain your current position will be obsolete in five to seven years. The body of knowledge in your profession may double every two or three years.

About 70 percent of working people feel "used up" at day's end, and half describe themselves as "highly stressed." More than 25 percent of us—right now—have stress-induced illnesses.

Stress can suppress your immune system, making you susceptible to infectious diseases—viruses such as flu or bacterial infections such as pneumonia. Stress causes the heart to beat quicker, which makes you vulnerable to chest pain (angina) and irregular heart rhythms. Stress may even lead to heart attack or stroke. We have each heard of someone dying of a broken heart.

Stress is indeed a health issue, and who isn't stressed today?

My point? The workplace is changing. These profound changes affect our health, and the workplace is where the effects of health are so obvious. Today's workforce is mobile. Your current employer has little vested interest in keeping you healthy over the long term so you'll live longer and healthier because, chances are, you won't be working at that company in your later years when all the prevention measures you could take now start to payoff in terms of longevity. In fact, you may be a liability to your employer if you collect on retirement plans or remain on a company's health insurance plan because you're living longer and healthier. They'd rather you didn't stick around.

Work itself contributes to stress. Service-with-a-smile takes a toll. Those of you engaged in "emotional labor" know all too well the incredible strain on your mental and physical abilities. Emotional labor refers to the process of controlling emotions that is required by service workers, such as retail sales associates, administrative assistants, flight attendants, customer care representatives, telemarketers, and others who are expected to cope with difficult customers and clients.

Demanding interactions can result in negative mental and physical health, says a Penn State researcher. "Service with a smile, especially when mandated by a company, may be pleasing to the customer, but at the same time, it may be emotionally and physically stressful for the employee, especially if forced or insincere," said Alicia A. Grandey, associate professor of psychology. "Job stress does more than cause absenteeism, decreased productivity, fatigue, and burnout. The physiological bottling-up of emotions taxes the body over time by overworking the cardiovascular and nervous systems, and weakening the immune system."

If you're in one of these service-with-a-smile positions, and difficult customers start to get to you, learn to redirect your emotional response. I encourage you to take a brief walk, begin deep-breathing exercises, or try internal self-talk that allows you to reappraise a bad experience with a customer—especially if your employer doesn't have similar debriefing strategies.

What's your alternative? A job with few responsibilities and no customer contact? Mindless jobs, on one hand, might sound attractive to the stressed-out, battle-worn workers. But think again. Working Americans with little opportunity for decision making die earlier than those with more flexibility, even if those flexible jobs are also high-stress positions.

The lack of control you have in your job may predict your death. In other words, if you have little control over your job, you are more likely to have stress-related problems caused by work than employees who have high-stress jobs but more decision-making responsibilities.

Meaningfulness of work, then, like meaningfulness in life, can make a difference in your health. In the 1940s, an Austrian-born psychiatrist, Dr. Viktor Frankl, was imprisoned in a concentration camp during the Holocaust. He survived an incredibly soul-shredding experience and tried to discern why some survived and some died. He made the observation that prisoners who had a reason to live, who had a "why" to live, somehow crafted the "how" to live. In other words, meaning and purpose somehow gave them the will to survive.

How do we find meaning and purpose in what we do?

There are no easy answers, but the long-term survivors in science, in business, and in a variety of professions seem to have the following characteristics, and I discuss this in more detail in the last chapter of this book:

- Survivors have their health. If our health goes south, nothing else matters. Just think about the last time you had surgery, the flu, an infection, or an injury in a serious car crash. The last thing you thought about was your investment portfolio or your projects at work. And those who lose their health can still maintain a sense of "wellness." Think about it. "Health" and "wellness" are two quite different states. For example, someone with a major disability may not be physically healthy but is certainly "well" in a powerful sense. Whereas an Olympic athlete— the epitome of physical health—could be a child abuser and not "well" at all.
- Survivors have a sense of community, a sense of connectedness. They somehow bond with colleagues, and a common task can generate a communal energy, which is greater than any single individual can generate.
- Survivors always have a sense of challenge; they never become complacent. I became intrigued with entertainers Siegfried and Roy, for example. I asked them how they performed the same Las Vegas show thousands of times, on a grueling schedule physically and mentally. Each responded that he always tried to make it perfect—fully recognizing that the show can never be perfect. This kept them going night after night, performance after performance, week after week, because they loved what they did. When tragedy struck in the form of a white tiger attack on Roy, they were mentally and physically capable of coping.
- Survivors always look for new challenges and new opportunities, and face each day as a gift and as a promise.

How Does Your Body Say, "I'm Stressed"?

Keeping your internal stress a secret is not easy. Stressed-out people do a number of incredibly annoying things with their bodies. Business communications expert Barbara Pachter points out that it's what you *don't* say that says a lot about you. She has listed the top 10 nonverbal cues that say "I'm stressed" in her book *The Power of Positive Confrontation*:

1. Point finger at others
2. Stick out tongue/lick lips when speaking
3. Wring hands
4. Sway
5. Use very stern facial expression
6. Use too broad or no gestures at all/hands on hips
7. Pound fist
8. Tap foot when seated
9. Look at floor when speaking
10. Play with change in pocket

Check these behaviors at your next employee meeting, and see if you can spot who's stressed. Let's hope it's not you.

It's About Time

These days, time management is not optional. Without it, stress levels would really be out of control. A revered cardiologist, Dr. Robert Eliot, said, "Manage your time as if your life depended on it ... because it does."

The average American is working more than 50 hours a week and has become enslaved by fiber optics. Yet none of these so-called labor-saving devices or technologies—computer, tablet, smartphone, e-mail—has really saved any time whatsoever. Time has become a noose around our collective necks. Laboratory animals bombarded by uncontrollable stimuli like this are not happy campers. And neither are we.

How many messages do you get every working day? Let's call them interruptions. These interruptions include telephone calls, voice mails, texts, reminders from your electronic planner, beepers, e-mail messages—and all require a response. How often are you checking your devices? Is your smartphone glued to your hand? Wonder why your neck hurts (from looking down)? Or why your thumbs are painful (from texting)? These are some of the new ailments caused by our electronic devices.

The landline phone may not ring as much, but your smartphone is dinging all day with incoming texts and e-mails. A Harris Interactive survey said most people can handle about 50 messages a day. After that, the respondents said they can't keep up. How many of those 90 trillion e-mails flying through the air in any given year are targeting you?

Trying to get your work done while being interrupted by technology only makes you less able to accomplish any tasks. No wonder we're stressed and can't get anything done.

If we permit interruptions, we're making one of the five worst mistakes of time management. The other four mistakes of time management are these:

- Spending time on issues that are not your priority, but someone else's "stuff"
- Underestimating the time a task consumes (because nothing is simple)
- Saying "yes" without thinking
- Not asking for help

A fascinating book in this regard is Winifred Gallagher's *Rapt: Attention and the Focused Life*. Drawing upon the experience of other experts, behavioral science writer Gallagher indicates that if we are interrupted in a task, on balance, it may take up to 15 minutes to recover and get back to where we were.

Let me elaborate on this point. I recently addressed a wonderful audience of engineers at the IBM campus here in Rochester, Minnesota. When I commented about the threat of interruptions, an IBM engineer shared with me the following story.

Several years ago, he became the lead engineer on a mission-critical function to help IBM survive some of the changes in the technology world. About 10 to 12 assistant engineers were freed up from other responsibilities and tasked to develop and bring to market a new type of computer. Their workday was organized so that collectively they would hit the pause button at their workstations, have an update, and then they would reboot their computers. Therefore, it was easy to calculate where they were in the project, how long the interruption lasted, and how long it took for them to get up to speed.

Bottom line, the results were fascinating. The amount of time to get back to where they were to get the job done was a doubling of the time of the interruption. So if there is a knock at your door and someone asks for 10 minutes of time, it will take you on average 20 minutes to get back to where you were.

The take-home message is clear: If there is a mission-critical function at work and at home—something that you need to do to get a job done—you must turn off the smartphone, the tablet, the computer, and focus on the task or it will never get appropriately done.

Gallagher also offers commentary that the length of time of maximum concentration is approximately 90 minutes. Occasionally, if we are rested and focused, we might push it to 120 minutes (2 hours), but without a break and some diversion, we start to spin our wheels and read, and reread, the same sentence multiple times.

One place to win the time-management battle is the dreaded "meeting." Realistically, most meetings are held for historical or informational purposes only. Little is accomplished. A Harvard Business School study says 90 percent of meetings accomplish very little. Meanwhile, you're sitting there, and time is tick, tick, ticking away. If you're in a position to make it happen, insist on an agenda and prompt start and stop times. Otherwise, you're wasting everyone's time.

Delegation is another winner in the time-management equation. No one individual can meet the needs of an organization. Each of us at the start of the day has so many units of energy. We must decide how to prioritize time and talents, or someone else will. Constructive delegation of responsibility frees us to focus on important tasks and to empower other individuals.

You may have heard this story or read a forwarded version of this unattributed Internet wisdom, but indulge me as I retell it in my own way.

When is your jar full?

A philosophy professor stood before the class with a large empty mayonnaise jar and proceeded to fill it with big rocks. He then asked students if the jar was full. They agreed it was.

So the professor picked up a box of pebbles and poured them into the jar. He shook the jar lightly. The pebbles, of course, rolled into the open areas between the rocks.

"Is the jar full now?" he asked.

The students agreed the jar was full. The professor picked up a box of sand and poured it into the jar. Of course, the sand filled up everything else.

"*Now*," said the professor, "I want you to recognize that this is your life. The rocks are the important things—your family, your partner, your health, your children—things that if everything else was lost and only they remained, your life would still be full.

"The pebbles are the other things that matter, like your job, your house, your car," he said.

"The sand is everything else. The small stuff."

Because this was a philosophy class, the professor went on to explain: "If you put the sand (the small stuff) into the jar first, there is no room for the pebbles or the rocks (the important things in life). The same goes for your life. If you spend all your time and energy on the small stuff, you will never have room for the things that are important to you.

"Pay attention to the things that are critical to your happiness. Play with your children. Take time to get medical checkups. Take your partner out dancing. There will always be time to go to work, clean the house, give a dinner party, and fix the disposal. Take care of the rocks first—the things that really matter. Set your priorities. The rest is just sand."

Examine what you have in your mayonnaise jar. Are you sweating the pebbles—the small stuff—or the sand? Or do you make time to put the rocks in first?

Of course, this delightful (albeit apocryphal) story came over the Internet, and it continues. A student took the jar, which all had agreed was quite full, and poured a glass of beer into it. The moral is that there's always room for beer, but this is a book about prevention, so I don't recommend adding beer.

I divide time (the rocks, pebbles and sand of life) into the following types:

- **Prime time.** These are those hours (or minutes) of the day when your energy can be focused like a heat-seeking missile. No interruptions. If you're working, this is the work time when you're at your peak. For me, it's the early morning hours. Again, most experts suggest that we are at our peak for no more than 90 to 120 minutes. Tackle your hardest work when you are the sharpest. Your enthusiasm during this time has a targeted velocity. Guard this time with the intensity of a Rottweiler. Do not give it away. This is your hour of power. Turn off the electronic devices and shut down incoming e-mail and social network surfing.
- **Brain-stem time.** Use this for mechanical, mundane chores such as sorting out junk mail, signing routine correspondence, and minding other mindless burdens that can be effectively dispatched during this time.
- **Away time.** These are precious occasions when we are physically removed from the arena and can direct our energies to tasks of renewal. We golf, garden, run, paint— these activities revive body and soul. Away time allows us to remove the yoke for a short time and know that we do not have to save the world, at least for today. In other words, leave the Wi-Fi devices at home, or you might as well be at the office. Sad but true, a laptop ad in *The Wall Street Journal* says it well: "The good news is that you're always connected to the office. The bad news is that you're always connected to the office."

In planning your time, it's preferable to avoid time leaks. Phone calls, e-mail, and texts can quickly become enormous time-wasters and block your coronary arteries. They do not save time. Try to handle routine inquiries between specific hours. Return messages just before lunch and just before you leave for the day. Stand while you return phone calls. They tend to be shorter. If you work at home, separate home and office. It's difficult but necessary.

Research has shown that messages responded to at these planned times are typically shorter. Keep pen in hand to complete uncomplicated paperwork so that time spent waiting on hold or waiting for a web page to download is not completely wasted.

Create Your Psychological Moat

One of the most important times in time management (and stress reduction) is what I call the psychological "moat." This is a buffer of time between commitments. Transition time, in other words. This is the zone in which we switch gears to psychologically prepare for the next challenge. But how many of us grab files and dash into meetings or to the next customer, without readying our minds for the next mental challenge? We certainly wouldn't show up for the tennis or golf match or run the marathon of our lifetime just a few minutes before the event.

1. **Do not spend time on issues that are not your priority.** That means making a list in the morning or in the prior evening so you can do what is important to you that day. Otherwise, your work culture will siphon off your time and you'll go home feeling frustrated and unfulfilled and dream (have nightmares) about an overflowing inbox.

2. **Nothing is simple.** Everything takes three times longer than expected, so never underestimate the time something will take.

3. **If you say "yes" to interruptions, you are giving away a piece of your soul.** Turning off the pager, turning off the e-mail and texts, and turning off your computer may help save your life.

4. **If you continually say "yes" to everything, you in effect are saying "yes" to nothing.** We have so many units of energy in the morning, and if we do not determine how we use them, they will quickly evaporate like the early morning dew.

Don't like the movie? Rewrite the script!

I'm a list maker. I plan the week, not just the day. And I plan away time for each day or evening (a run, time in the gym, piano practice). If I write down the tasks, I greatly increase the chance they'll get done. And it puts me in the driver's seat. Checking things off my list is empowering. Try it.

Our response to stress is highly individual. But generally it's like a football player who has repetitive head trauma or knee trauma in the game. One hit, and he'll survive. But add up week after week of hits in a season, and he'll be hurting. He won't be able to handle it anymore. Same with concussions. The damage is cumulative.

Are you taking too many hits? Feeling too stressed? Here are five telltale signs:

1. You feel irritable.
2. You have sleep problems (you're either sleepy all the time or can't sleep).
3. You experience no joy. Life is a grind.
4. You develop a severe loss of appetite, or you can't stop eating.
5. You have trouble with relationships and no longer get along well with friends and family members.

It's all about attitude. Your outlook on life, in fact, may not only help you live longer, but it also appears to have an impact on your quality of life. Those of us who see the glass half full (the optimists) report a higher level of physical and mental functioning than those who see the glass half empty and don't look on the bright side of life (the pessimists). A study of lung cancer patients documents that those with nonpessimistic coping styles lived far longer than the pessimists. One of my colleagues has looked at the half-full glass, and his research is showing that outlook on life may help extend it.

"The wellness of being is not just physical, but attitudinal," said Dr. Toshihiko Maruta, lead author of the study published in *Mayo Clinic Proceedings*. "How you perceive what goes on around you and how you interpret it may have an impact on your longevity, and it could affect the quality of your later years."

Study participants were surveyed with a personality test in the 1960s, and again 30 years later. This is one of the first studies to report the long-term health effects of self-reported outlook. This study showed that if we can see a light at the end of the tunnel, we can also see a positive good, regardless of the circumstances. There's no question that to some extent we can determine our reality. We can learn to focus on what we have rather than on what we don't have.

For my cancer patients, this is rock solid. I can tell who's an optimist, and who is not, the moment I walk into the exam room. The distinction is startling.

Even with heart disease, a sense of optimism seems to protect health. Based on a scoring system that placed a group of men on a scale from pessimist to optimist, each step up the scale toward optimism decreased their risk of coronary heart disease. The most optimistic men had a risk of heart disease less than half of that for the most grouchy of the old men, according to a study headed by a Harvard researcher in the journal *Psychosomatic Medicine*.

The men were drawn from a group of veterans in their 60s who were followed for an average of 10 years. The researchers suggest that the protective effects of optimism may be, in part, caused by lower stress, which has been shown to decrease heart-disease risk. Also, the optimists in the study were more likely to engage in health-promoting activities, such as exercise, and not be smokers.

The researchers caution that the results are specific only to the study group, but let's be optimistic and say that stress management and having a healthy outlook on life certainly can't hurt.

Also, simple, cost-effective treatment can help people with diabetes control blood sugar, and I'm not talking about insulin shots. It's about stress management. A smile a day can keep the doctor away, in certain circumstances. Stress can increase glucose levels in people with diabetes, making them more susceptible to long-term physical complications, such as eye, kidney, blood vessel, or nerve disorders. In the short term, uncontrolled stress may lead to the release of hormones that activate the fight-or-flight response, dumping glucose into the bloodstream, which poses a health threat for someone with diabetes.

A research study at Duke University Medical Center focused on participants with type 2 diabetes who were taught how to identify everyday life stressors and how to respond to them, with such techniques as progressive muscle relaxation, mental imagery, and breathing exercises.

The researchers were able to show that these stress-management techniques, when added to standard care, helped reduce glucose levels, as much as might be expected with control drugs alone.

The only way to survive our stressful existence is to recognize that we have choices and options in the way we live and respond to stress. Let me offer 16 proven ways to reduce stress:

1. Simplify your life. Cut out some activities or delegate tasks. Use the extra time to relax. Use such exercises as controlling your breathing, clearing your mind, and relaxing your muscles.
2. View negative situations as positive and a chance to improve your life. What can I learn from this situation?
3. Use humor to reduce or relieve tension.
4. Exercise. It relieves tension and provides a "time out" from stressful situations: 30 minutes 5 days a week. Small investment.
5. Go to bed earlier. More sleep makes you stronger and more able to handle day-to-day life.
6. Reduce or eliminate caffeine. Caffeine is a stimulant.
7. Get a massage.
8. Keep a stress journal. Track what "sets you off," and learn to prioritize tasks. Do what is most important first.
9. Enjoy yourself. Read a good book or see an uplifting movie.
10. Take a hot bath.
11. Call a friend, and strengthen or establish a support network. Make the most of friends and family.
12. Set aside personal time. Limit time spent with "negative" people.
13. Hug your family and friends and pets.
14. Do volunteer work or start a hobby. Take a language course or pick up a guitar or piano. No, not physically lift the piano! When I was 62, with absolutely no musical background (and perhaps no ability either), I started piano lessons. Now, eight years later, I play one of the magnificent pianos on the Mayo campus for pure

enjoyment. My piano teacher has advised me to keep my medical license updated because I'm not ready for prime time.

15. Take a vacation. Take a day or longer to rejuvenate yourself.

16. Unplug from the gadgets that drive us nuts. Get off the grid. Have a screen-free day.

These quick, simple techniques to manage stress can often do more than my colleagues and I can do for you with medication.

Although there is little credible evidence that stress causes cancer, stress certainly can make your life miserable. It seems most reasonable to make all appropriate efforts to keep life at a reasonable level of chaos.

Resilience in the face of adversity

In the world of horse racing—a world my father knew too well—there is no such thing as luck. In fact, my father said this frequently. Let's look at the Kentucky Derby. It was 2005. A horse named Giacomo was hopelessly blocked behind a wall of horses with 3/16 of a mile to go. At 50 to 1 odds, the horse was disrespected by the betting public.

Minutes later, the most surprised person—or should I say "creature"—on the planet was Giacomo, who won the victory under the professional ride of jockey Mike Smith. Now let's talk about Mr. Smith, because this is not a story about a horse.

Approximately six years before Smith won the Kentucky Derby on Giacomo, he had taken a wicked spill at the Saratoga track in upstate New York. He had multiple vertebral compression fractures and almost became paralyzed. He was in a body cast for several weeks and knew that his fitness would be tragically deteriorating. He had the foresight and insight not to simply sit back, but hired and brought on board strength and conditioning coaches, dietitians, and other health care providers. He became proactive and preemptive because he knew that his greatest gift, as with each of us, is the gift of our health and well-being. After all, if our health deteriorates, nothing else really matters.

Nothing else mattered that day at the Derby when Smith rode to victory, albeit a long shot, in more ways than one. Luck had no effect here. And Mike Smith has continued a successful career having won some major races over the past year. His fitness routines are legendary at the track. I'm also talking about resiliency and drive.

Consider Mick Jagger. Talk about a durable performer who keeps up in the face of aging and adversity. The world's greatest rock-and-roll band continues to be the Rolling Stones, and according to *USA Today*, for 50 years they have continued to "cement their relevance." Their lifestyles have been criticized, but over the years, Jagger has continued to perform at an incredibly punishing pace with a daunting schedule.

The entertainment columns report that he lifts weights and does yoga and ballet. He follows a whole-grain, low-fat diet. So his durability may have less to do with luck and chance and much more to do with preparation and resiliency to maximize his performing skills.

Doctors and other health care professionals burn out. I see it all the time among my colleagues. Some are emotionally exhausted at times, and, sadly, others see an erosion of empathy with their patients. Doctors and nurses just can't bear their burdens any longer. They can become emotionally drained at the end of the day, which leads to career-ending events. Or death from stress-magnified illness such as heart disease.

Long work hours, on-call schedules, endless paperwork that's now also electronic, plus changes in health care reform and the uncertainties of Medicare and Medicaid all add to the burden health care providers face, and these burdens contribute to stress. Add to all this the frustrations of trying to navigate a cumbersome electronic medical record. These internal and external stress factors were examined in a physician survey, which revealed that nearly 87 percent of physicians are moderately to severely stressed.

Dr. Neil Rudenstine was a respected academician and the President of Harvard. Yet he appeared on the cover of *Newsweek* in 1995 as an example of exhaustion and burnout, all because he did not follow a number of simple rules. He did not have the gift to say no. He was burning the candle at both ends and did not recognize the importance of sleep, exercise, and appropriate nutrition. He had lost that ability to delegate and sort out what was really important.

While on our palliative care/hospice service several months ago I was working with a new resident physician—an energetic, creative woman in her early 30s. We met with seven different families in a row. These are emotionally heavy consultations because the loved one is in our intensive-care unit and facing possible end of life. There is always discussion of discontinuing respirator care, and that's a nice way to say, "Pull the plug."

We talk. Most important, we listen. We advise. Families are making soul-shredding decisions.

I asked my colleague how she was anticipating doing this kind of work day after day for the next 30 years, as I have done and continue to do, and she shared with me a powerful notion of resilience. In so many words, she basically said that after she walks out of the room, writes her notes, confers with other colleagues, and closes the computer on that patient, she also symbolically puts that patient out of her mind. Not in a disrespectful manner, but she acknowledges that she must flip that switch and move on because if she becomes embedded in the suffering of that patient and family, she will never be able to function. She uses the technique of compartmentalizing these dreadful events.

These types of compartmentalizing skills are like the pitcher who serves up a home run at a crucial point in the game, or a field goal kicker who misses. Like you, these people must develop a very short memory or they will never be able to function effectively under stress.

As a cancer specialist and as a palliative medicine hospice care physician, I know that this is a high-risk profession, and we must take care of ourselves. Here's a story that came to me recently.

On our campus, we are now building one of the largest integrated medical construction projects in Mayo Clinic history. This is the proton beam facility. One of our safety officers shared with me somewhat facetiously that it's probably safer to work on this construction project than to be a medical provider! How right he is.

As I walked by the worksite one day, I was struck by the overarching emphasis on safety. There were clearly marked signs that this was a tobacco-free and alcohol-free environment. Workers had to register.

They needed to have construction-grade helmets, protective goggles, knee and ankle and wrist guards, and also protective rigging. Safety and welfare were clearly ingrained into the DNA of the worker (and OSHA has some say here too). This was palpable, and the results were remarkable. Very few hours are lost to injury (as of this writing, over 600 days without an accident).

We in medicine and also in the corporate world sometimes don't recognize the hazards of where we work. Do we need psychological goggles and emotional helmets? Yes, in some ways, we do.

Wide awake at 3:00 a.m.

Another dimension that we cannot escape is the crushing impact of sleep deprivation. I'm reminded of a tragic commuter airplane crash outside of Buffalo, New York, several years ago, taking the lives of 50 people. An analysis of the pilot and copilot found that each was sleep deprived.

Some of my closest friends are airline captains, and I have often asked them to tell me what they have learned about sleep deprivation. They emphasize that our ability to perform complex tasks starts to dramatically deteriorate after approximately 17 hours of wakefulness. So let's think about this. If you are up at 5:00 a.m., as is typical with many of us, spend a full day with work or activities, return home, help the kids with the homework, prepare the meals, clean up the dishes, and pay some bills, by the time you get to bed, it's 10:00 p.m.—and there are your 17 hours of wakefulness. You need sleep. You don't want to be wide awake at 3:00 a.m.

Three of the greatest human-related disasters of the past several decades all occurred at approximately 3:00 a.m.: the Three Mile Island nuclear leak, the crash and devastating oil spill of the *Exxon Valdez*, and the Chernobyl nuclear accident.

Consider this, if your wakefulness includes the hours of either 3:00 a.m. to 5:00 a.m., as is the case for shift workers, that's the second concern about fatigue. If your sleep is fragmented or interrupted so that you are not getting seven solid hours of sleep, you are clinically functioning at a level equal to being legally drunk. And you don't even know it.

On a Sunday morning in 1980, the Miracle on Ice took place. A group of college kids, primarily from Minnesota, as part of the Olympics took on one of the greatest hockey teams in the history of the sport: the Russian Red Army team. Herb Brooks was the coach of the American team—a beloved, iconic sports figure in the state of Minnesota. With keen coaching insight and punishing conditioning, the American kids beat the Russians and came home with the gold medal.

Several summers ago, Mr. Brooks returned to Minnesota for some social activities. He was tragically killed in a single car accident on a bright sunny day, with no evidence of drugs or alcohol or even skid marks. Authorities suspected that he simply fell asleep at the wheel, so perhaps his busy schedule had something to do with his sleep deprivation.

The lesson is this: you need sleep. Your body needs sleep. It's as important as eating and breathing.

And when it comes to eating, a sleepless night might even make you reach for donuts or pizza, suggest researchers at University of California–Berkeley, who looked at brain regions that control food choices. Lack of sleep, they said, shuts down high-level brain regions required for you to make complex decisions, such as choosing a whole-grain bread for a sandwich over a greasy pizza. Your brain on less sleep craves sweet and salty foods, not an apple. The researchers speculate that sleep deprivation plays a role in obesity.

No, you can't multitask

Very simply and directly, as much as you think you can, you cannot multitask. Never mind walking and chewing gum, you cannot neurologically or physiologically do two things at once. Well, actually you *can* walk and chew gum, because one is a thinking task and one is a nonthinking task. Whereas, driving and talking on a cell phone are two thinking tasks, and the brain can't do both at once, so says the National Safety Council, among others.

People who try to drive and text or talk are toggling back and forth between each function. During the time it takes to rewire the brain, a tragic accident can happen. Distracted driving accidents are happening everywhere.

Not only am I advising you not to try to drive and text or talk on the phone, or even walk and text or drive, I am advising you to watch out for the "other guys" who think they can. I said sleep deprivation is like being legally drunk. Well, driving and talking on a cell phone (even hands-free talking makes no difference) is even worse than being legally drunk. Reactions times are slower.

Distracted driving accounts for 7.3 million people running red lights per year, according to the National Coalition for Safer Roads. That inattentive driver yakking away about the grocery list could be headed right toward you or your loved ones at any intersection anywhere.

Distractions will interfere with the performance of routine tasks. Here's an example: Several years ago, a gentleman from a major city awoke on a Sunday morning with severe left flank pain. He had chills, fever and sweats, and wine-colored urine (like a cabernet). His primary care provider was appropriately concerned about a condition called "pyelonephritis" or an infection of the kidney. Even worse news, a CT scan showed an obvious cancer in the left kidney.

The patient had superb preoperative assessments, and surgery went smoothly. However, a routine postoperative CT scan was shocking. What doctors saw was this: the left kidney was fully intact with the cancer, and the patient's healthy, cancer-free right kidney was missing.

This was absolute devastation for everyone involved in the patient's care, as well as for the patient and the family. A newspaper article chronicling these tragic events indicated that the surgeon, distracted by beeper calls and other interruptions, made a tragic mistake in the operating room.

So we need to recognize that we have limits and cannot continuously push the envelope.

Shoelaces and stress

We've all seen pictures of the newly appointed CEO when he or she enters the corporate boardroom with a youthful bounce and an adolescent vitality, with all the gifts, skills, and charm to turn around a failing organization. What about the press conference introducing the new coach appointed to revive a losing athletic team? How does he or she look several years after being on the corporate or athletic or academic treadmill?

Haggard. Wrinkled. Less hair, and certainly less joy. These people undergo a dramatic physical change, a physical transformation clearly precipitated by the crushing burdens of responsibility. Now is this just the way it is, or can we learn some important lessons from this experience? How can we ourselves go the distance when faced with real challenges?

Let's think back to high school biology. We all vaguely remember that our genetic material is housed in pieces of DNA called chromosomes. These are structures that look like two horseshoes joined at their round ends, and all of our characteristics in terms of height and weight and intelligence and flexibility and eye color are determined by these little capsules of genetic information. The ends of these capsules contain some proteins that are called telomeres. These are much like the plastic caps on the ends of shoelaces.

We've all had the frustration of having these plastic caps break off when lacing our shoes. Then not even a skillful surgeon can thread the shoelace into the eye of the shoe. Now these telomeres are far more important than our shoelaces. These are the caps that keep our genetic material from unraveling or unrolling. When these telomeres become shortened or deformed and do not work effectively, the genetic material becomes rearranged, fragmented, and when it joins back together again, it creates a mutant state—and the results might not be what we anticipate.

The mutant genetic material may clearly give rise to heart disease, cancer, strokes, and all sorts of miseries. So what does this interesting biological event have to do with us? Well, it has a lot to do with us.

Fascinating studies examined the telomeres of women who cared for their developmentally disabled children. This was a 24/7/365 commitment with virtually no reprieve. These mothers were heroic, but they had limits and they became fatigued and drained and completely overwhelmed with the demands of these youngsters.

They also recognized that at no point would these children become independent and self-sufficient.

Measurements of the telomeres of the stressed women provided a dramatic result. These protective end caps were far smaller, far shorter than in individuals who were relatively comfortable and did not have the crushing burden of caring for these children. There is also evidence that, with stress reduction techniques and other interventions that I mention in this book, the telomeres can be restored to their previous levels of integrity. In other words, some stress-management techniques can put the "end caps" back onto the shoelaces.

There's also evolving evidence that yoga, meditation, mindfulness, times of thoughtful introspection and silence and solitude can enhance the functioning of these protective caps on our genetic material. So the stage is set. There are things that we can do to lessen stress.

Here is the *Reader's Digest* version of what we can do to maintain the functional capacity of these telomeres:

Be mindful of the role of stress in your life. It's not simply the fact that you become irritable, short tempered, don't sleep, and may struggle with heart disease and depression; the consequences are far more significant in terms of rearranging and damaging your genetic material. A good night's sleep. Making a list. Having clear boundaries and priorities. All these are obvious steps in the right direction. What do we need to do for ourselves today?

You've heard the mantra a million times, "Use it or lose it." And this really applies to the role of physical activity in maintaining the thickness of these telomeres. The usual recommendation of at least 30 minutes of aerobic activity most days is absolutely crucial to maintaining health and well-being.

We all have been advised to eat plenty of fruits and vegetables, but we also have to recognize the overarching protective effect of whole grains, such as in breads and cereals, that can enhance the telomere length. Colored fruits and vegetables, green leafy fruits and vegetables containing vitamins E and C also protect telomeres from the damage of oxidative metabolism. Nutrients found naturally in fruits and vegetables are far more beneficial and far more available to us than the ones we obtain from taking supplements.

As a little boy, I remember my grandmother with her Irish brogue encouraging me to eat fish because it was "brain food." I'm not certain I'm any smarter because I followed her advice, but, unbeknownst to me and certainly unbeknownst to my grandmother, the omega-3 fatty acids in fish decrease inflammation and oxidative metabolism and help protect our telomeres.

So we are again hearing the same theme. This is not brain surgery. This is not rocket science. This isn't even high school calculus.

Now, of course, some conditions are genetically determined, and we have no control over them. I'm speaking of certain types of inherited cancers and certain types of neurologic and muscular disorders. However, for the vast majority of us, we can clearly put our hands on the helm of health, and the spokes of that helm are the kinds of lifestyle choices and options that we have addressed.

Strength through stress

You can buffer some of the slings and arrows that assault you every day. Because you are the author of your life, you can change the script and handle the stress of life more effectively. Let me offer some ideas:

- **Find joy in life.** Develop a genuine commitment to something that gives you great pleasure. Keep your passion going, whether it's coaching your child's soccer team, rummaging around old bookstores, or collecting butterflies. Find time for relaxation. Clear your mind. Start with small chunks of time for yourself. Find things you enjoy outside of work and other obligations—paint, dance, take a course at a community college. Block off time each day for the "joy."
- **Face challenges.** View difficulties as challenges to confront and master, rather than as situations to flee from. Learn to see life as a challenge and opportunity, even in your darkest moments. Most of us get frustrated with mistakes and failure when things don't work. Expect things not to work. When something fails, you might even think: *See, I told you, it wouldn't work.* Anticipate outcomes and ask yourself up front: *What if it doesn't work?* Don't let your

decisions weigh you down like a rock around your neck. Figure out what you learned from the experience, and move on. Repeat after me: Move on. It's not worth it!

- **Control what you can.** Focus on what you do have control over, not what you don't. When life is screaming along at 200 miles per hour and seems out of control, what can you do to put the brakes on? Create boundaries between home and work, or between you and other obligations such as caregiving.

- **Laugh.** The antidote to stress may just be laughter. If you're looking forward to a favorite comedy on TV, just checking the TV listings may trigger healthy mood changes, reduce your stress hormone levels, and boost your immune system's defenses. A study presented at a Society for Neuroscience meeting was the first to show that anticipation of a mirthful event may be good for you. Dr. Lee Berk, associate professor at Loma Linda University, found that anticipating a laugh-inducing event reduced levels of tension, anger, depression, fatigue, and confusion up to two days before the actual event.

  "We've demonstrated that watching a funny video can stimulate the body's ability to manage stress and fight disease," Dr. Berk said, referring to his research on the mood-enhancing effects of comedy, which he has dubbed *laughercise*. "But this is the first time we've seen that just anticipating such an event can change the body's responses. We believe this 'biology of hope' underlies recovery from many chronic disorders."

So how do we summarize all of this information? I recommend you read a life-changing book, if you haven't discovered it already, entitled *The Last Lecture* (by Dr. Randy Pausch with Jeffrey Zaslow). Dr. Pausch had been on the top of his personal and professional game. He was a tenured professor at Carnegie Mellon, a prestigious institution in Pennsylvania, but then his life tragically took a turn when he was diagnosed with advanced cancer of the pancreas. His book became an instant hit, and his YouTube videos and presentations on *Oprah* were spellbinding.

It's difficult to capture in a few moments the essence of his message, but let me try to do so:

1. He concentrated on what was really important. I can recall one scene in the book where there was some frustration in a checkout line where he may have been overcharged a few dollars. Ordinarily, he would have spoken to the manager and spent a lot of time on this issue, but he knew that the clock was ticking, and he was not willing to spend time on the issue of the few dollars. As Ben Franklin said, "Time lost is never found again."

2. He clearly stressed the importance of connections. The power of his parents in his life and the energy and the support he garnered from his wife and children were immeasurable—and what life was all about.

3. He stressed physical conditioning to maximize his dealing with cancer. In fact, on *Oprah* he easily performed several dozen push-ups effortlessly.

Get a life—connectedness can happen

Study after study has documented that a sense of community, a sense of connectedness, and a life partner to whom we can cling in times of stress, all may be measurable and workable solutions to finding sanity in the midst of chaos.

Here's how.

You've told your teenagers to "get a life" a million times when they sleep until noon and leave their dirty laundry around as if it will magically turn into folded, clean stacks. They act as if the world revolves around them. We're all teenagers in the sense that we all want the world to revolve around us, but what really works wellness-wise is getting out into the world and getting connected.

Connectedness can happen; we all want to be connected, to widen our social circle throughout life, not just at a time of crisis or illness. Let me offer some tried-and-true ways to do that:

- **Volunteer.** Studies have shown that older people who stay connected to others by volunteering live longer than those who don't volunteer. Certainly, your local hospital can use your help, but so can schools. Read with elementary students. Tutor at a nearby high school. Visit someone who's caring for an ailing relative or friend. Serve lasagna at a homeless shelter. Offer your services to organizations that help victims of domestic violence. Usher at the theater. Deliver meals to the elderly. Drive disabled veterans to the VA Medical Center. Become a foster family, or be a dog walker for your animal shelter. Work at the food bank. Give blood.

- **Share your knowledge.** Are you retired from law or business or sales? Hook up with organizations that assist new and small businesses. Teach gardening at the community college, or offer personal enrichment programs, such as quilting or picture framing, through your school district. If photography is your hobby, teach it. If you always loved coaching your kids (or never made time) and now they're grown, coach other people's kids.

- **Work at your hobby.** Go ahead and buy the '64 Chevy Super Sport and restore it in your garage. Set a goal and make it happen. Browse a craft fair and engage an avid crafter to find out how you can get started making candles, stringing beaded bracelets, or designing holiday ornaments. Scan Etsy and Pinterest for ideas. If you use your analytical left brain in your business and work life, maybe it's time to tap into the creative right side for better life balance.

- **Go back to school.** Learning is a lifelong activity. Take a class. Finish a degree. Earn college credit. Check out adult ed classes near you. Cooking and restaurant meal-tasting are popular, as are day trips to art museums and nearby historic sites. And look into MOOCs—these are massive open online courses taught by revered profs at prestigious universities. The online classes are open to anyone anywhere with an Internet connection. Oh, yes, they are absolutely free. Start at *Coursera.org*.

- **Get a pet.** If you choose a dog, you'll have a ready-made walking partner. But pets can work magic in other ways too: Teach your pet. Take your dog to obedience class. Or simply take your dog to the park, and enjoy Fido's ability to attract people.

- **Be a sport.** Attend local sporting events, such as college basketball, youth soccer, league hockey, peewee baseball. Ask if you can help. And by all means join a wellness center where you can exercise your mind, body, and spirit with others. Take the yoga class you always said you wanted to try.
- **Join something.** What interests you? Mystery writing? Duplicate bridge? Small engines? Cooking? Drumming? Tarot cards? Find a special interest group by scanning community calendars and online bulletin boards in your city, or create your own group by posting notices online (Craigslist) or in the grocery store. Meet regularly at a local bookstore or coffee shop.
- **Attend worship services.** Studies show that older people who attend religious services live longer than those who don't attend services. Church groups are always seeking volunteers and making social events out of raking leaves, painting houses for the disadvantaged, or conducting clothing drives.
- **And don't forget to ask people about themselves!** Each person you ask will become a friend for life.

My Balance Rx

Feeling too busy to take care of yourself? Not enough time to worry about diet and exercise or regular checkups? You'll have lots of down time in the intensive-care unit when your heart decides to give you a wake-up call. Think about it. If you don't have time to get gas for your car, you'll pay later for sure when you're at the side of the road. Same with your body.

One of the most important lessons in stress management is discovery of a sacred space where we can put on our emotional armor before heading back into the arena. This may be a stunning hiking trail in Glacier National Forest, a sweet fishing spot in the wilds of Northern Minnesota's Boundary Waters, or a sugar-sand beach lapped by warm turquoise water. Your escape may be virtual—a mental vacation using imagery to take you to your sacred place when you can't physically go there.

So what do I do and what have I learned about trying to deal with the stresses and the unfairness of life?

For the past 33 years, every April, I go on a silent retreat in the tradition of the Jesuits. This is a three-day program at a college campus-type environment just east of Minneapolis. I've been attending this program with the same group of approximately 40 men, some of whom have died over the years. Since it is silent, we really don't know much about each other. So we don't become distracted talking about the weather, sports, and politics. It is understood that this is a time for us to think, to pray, and to create an environment of introspection.

A recent study at the University of Michigan has confirmed that a nondenominational spiritual retreat can help patients with severe heart trouble feel less depressed and more hopeful about the future.

I'm reminded that almost every great spiritual thinker of both the Eastern and Western traditions has taken time from his or her public presence to go to the mountain, to go to the desert, to go to the sea, to go to the garden, to go to the sacred space for quiet time to renew the batteries and then go back into the turmoil of life—renewed, refreshed, recharged, with a new perspective on what is important and what is not.

Alcohol: Use Not Abuse

Some people should not drink alcohol. I'm one of them. After descending from four generations of alcoholics, I don't need to be told twice that alcohol and I simply won't mix. As the only son of two alcoholics, I know the risks and chose not ever to use alcohol. Others may enjoy a glass of red wine (just one) to avoid heart disease. But where alcohol use may spillover into abuse, moderation is the watchword. (In addition, alcohol can be harmful to many health conditions, including breast cancer.)

Most studies seem to suggest that at least 10 percent of the American population is chemically dependent. No one can calculate alcohol's full role in marital discord, fatal automobile accidents, and the ruin of productive and creative lives. If you or someone you love is concerned about alcoholism, this clearly requires the input of a credentialed professional.

Many of us in clinical medicine use the phrase "CAGE" to assess when use becomes abuse. Now what does this mean?

C: Have you ever felt a need to *cut* down on your drinking?

A: Do you become *annoyed* when someone comments about your drinking?

G: Have you ever felt *guilty* about drinking?

E: Do you require an "*eye* opener" to start the day, or are you drinking in the morning?

If an individual says yes to two or more of these four questions, we doctors raise a red flag about chemical dependency. (Yes to the E question alone is also a red flag.) The implications are far-reaching. A hallmark of alcoholism is denial, and it is difficult for the individual to be objective about his or her own drinking habits. That is why doctors need the input of family and community to help us determine the extent of a person's chemical dependency.

If someone you love and care about is abusing alcohol (or you think such abuse is occurring), seek help for yourself. A trained counselor can guide you in how to approach the situation.

Moderation may apply to alcohol use, but it does not apply to the next subject: smoking.

The No-Smoking Section

Here we are, 50 years after the U.S. Surgeon General Dr. Luther Terry released the first Surgeon General's report on smoking and health in 1964. Dr. Terry's 387-page report on the link between smoking and cancer and other serious diseases was released on a Saturday because reports say that President Lyndon Johnson was concerned that its contents would have an effect on the stock market.

This was the first official word from Washington on the cause-and-effect relationship between smoking and disease. Today, the official word is inscribed on every cigarette pack sold.

So where are we today? The tobacco industry has admitted blame. Smokers have a tough time finding a place to smoke in public. You can't smoke in restaurants or bars or workplaces (and some companies even ban smoking in your own vehicle in a company parking lot). Hotels and motels are smoke-free. Schools and college campuses and dorms are often smoke-free. Nobody smokes on airplanes or in airports, except in a few crowded, smoke-filled nooks. Cars don't even come with ashtrays.

Yet people still buy cigarettes, smoke them, and die.

Consider this. What if all cigarette smoking in this country had stopped following the release of Dr. Terry's report in 1964? A total of 2.5 million people would have been spared from death due to lung cancer in the years following that report, according to a study in the *Journal of the National Cancer Institute*. Maybe someone you knew. On the happier side, a Yale study in 2014 estimates that 8 million premature deaths have been avoided as a result of those antismoking measures.

Admittedly, cigarette smoking has been on the decline in the United States over the past 60-plus years, moving from a high of 45 percent in 1954 to 19 percent today, according to the CDC. (Who among us doesn't cringe while watching the popular TV show *Mad Men,* where the 1960s ad agency characters smoke openly in the office and just about everywhere else?)

Even so, today, 43.8 million adults smoke (with 4,000 teens joining those ranks every day). More men than women smoke.

Among all smokers, 69 percent would like to quit. Most smokers know it's harmful to themselves and others. They know it causes lung cancer, heart disease, and other ills. Two-thirds of smokers have tried to quit. So why don't they?

Tobacco industry insider, Jeffrey Wigand, Ph.D., the whistle-blower whose story was told in the movie *The Insider*, tells audiences across the country that cigarettes are the only product that "when used as intended, kill you." He looks nothing like the actor Russell Crowe, by the way, who played his role so brilliantly for Hollywood, but Dr. Wigand doesn't need glitz and glamour to make his points:

There is no "safe cigarette." But the tobacco industry is attempting to polish its image in the aftermath of the massive tobacco settlement by developing so-called safer products. The newer models may be lower in tar, but the extra baggage that comes along with the nicotine has four to eight times the amount of carbon monoxide than regular smokes. "If you want carbon monoxide," Dr. Wigand suggests, "go suck the exhaust of a school bus."

Although cigarettes are unregulated and require no ingredients label like foods do, the list of ingredients would include 599 different chemicals intended to maintain their hold on addicted smokers. Some of these ingredients are so toxic and carcinogenic (cancer-causing), you cannot dispose of them legally in this country—except through cigarettes.

To break the bonds of smoking's chemical and physical addiction, Dr. Wigand suggests nicotine-replacement therapy, plus medication and behavioral modification. This may require the guidance of a nicotine-dependency counselor. There are now several approved medications to help patients with this complex issue of addiction. Even at that, only half of people will be able to quit. Smokers often try five times before they become successful quitters.

The vast majority of lung cancers are directly related to cigarette smoking, even though a small minority of patients who never smoked will get lung cancer. If the cancer cannot be surgically removed, only a small percentage of patients are alive at five years after diagnosis. The average survival for patients with advanced lung cancer is less than a year.

Bladder cancer is yet another disease linked to smoking. Cigarette smokers are two to three times more likely than nonsmokers to get bladder cancer—the fourth most common cancer in men and the eighth most common among women. Nothing prevents these types of cancer better than not smoking at all—or quitting if you do smoke.

Safer alternatives?

Enter the electronic cigarette. Is it really a cigarette? No, it's a nicotine-delivery system. These devices have a battery-operated heating element. They look like cigarettes—or even everyday items like pens or memory sticks—and they deliver nicotine and other substances in the form of vapor. Users switch out the cartridges.

At this writing, the FDA has not evaluated any e-cigarettes for safety or effectiveness, but has noted issues with quality and inconsistent amounts of nicotine in similar cartridges. So far, up to 14 percent of smokers have adopted e-cigarettes.

Experts have, of course, raised concerns that the marketing of e-cigarettes can increase nicotine addiction among young people and may lead kids to try other tobacco products. With no-smoking laws banning smoking in most public places, the e-cigarette brings a certain appeal for smokers who really need a nicotine hit. So far, the jury is out on where e-cigarettes—whose manufacturers tout that they can be used "everywhere"—really can be used. Most airlines ban them, as do many hotels.

The devices do not emit secondhand smoke, but they do emit harmful chemicals into the air. Let's see where this all leads us, but certainly a cigarette by any other name is still harmful.

Instead of using e-cigarettes with their questionable and unproven ability to assist smokers in quitting, the FDA has approved smoking cessation aids, including nicotine gum, nicotine skin patches, nicotine lozenges, nicotine oral inhaled products, and nicotine nasal spray, all of which are available for smokers to use to reduce their dependence on nicotine. Your doctor can share the pros and cons of these options. A certified nicotine-dependency counselor is the ideal professional in this regard.

The allure of a fine cigar has shaped public perception and misinformation about them. The glamorous image of cigar smokers clouds the issue: The real issue is that cigar smoking, like cigarette smoking, is known to cause lung cancer. Rates of cigar smoking are rising among adults and adolescents (among both teenage boys and girls). Many see cigars as a safer alternative to cigarettes, but they are not.

Smoking cigars instead of cigarettes does not reduce the risk of nicotine addiction either. And the more you inhale, the more your risk of death related to cigar smoking increases—and may reach as high a risk level as that for smoking cigarettes.

Use of smokeless tobacco, either as dip (tobacco placed between the lip and gum) or chew (chewed tobacco), has increased among young white men who think, incorrectly, that it's a healthier choice than smoking cigarettes. Its use is strongly linked to cancer of the mouth, vocal cords—and everything else down to the stomach.

Marijuana use increases risk for head or neck cancers. Researchers from UCLA found that subjects in their study who had used marijuana were more than twice as likely to develop these deadly cancers. The more marijuana the subjects used, the greater their risk. Marijuana smoke contains as much as 50 percent higher concentrations of known cancer-causing substances and deposits four times as much tar in the respiratory tract as one cigarette does. Use of water pipes or hookahs is even more deadly.

Even hard-core smokers can quit

Imagine a research study of smokers who have smoked for an average of 22 years, most of whom have tried to quit in the past. They average more than a pack a day. Many have their first cigarette of the day within 15 minutes of waking up (an indicator that they are dependent on tobacco). That was the challenge in a study using nicotine gum plus tailored health messages. Bottom line: The combination of nicotine replacement and education was twice as likely to work—and helped longtime smokers quit for good.

"When a person decides to quit smoking by using nicotine-replacement therapy [this study used nicotine gum and was sponsored by its manufacturer], having personalized self-help materials … significantly improves their success," said a researcher who directs the Smoking Research Group at the University of Pittsburgh.

Smokers were given individualized information by mail based on their goals for quitting, their smoking history, their lack of success in quitting in the past, their target quit date, and the difficulties they expected. These tailored programs are often available through state smoking quit lines, through many employers (check with your HR/benefits department), and even from the pharmaceutical companies that make nicotine-replacement products. Use them.

Free help is also available to all smokers who want to quit. Call 1-800-QUIT-NOW, or visit *smokefree.gov*, a program administered by the NIH's National Cancer Institute.

It's hard for anyone to quit smoking, but women may have a tougher time, according to research reviewing several studies. Women and men have different issues when faced with the decision to quit.

Female smokers fear gaining a lot of weight if they quit; male smokers may fear this too, but to a far lesser degree. For men and women, the additional weight gain, if any, is far healthier than the damage the smoking is doing, even if smoking keeps off a few pounds. An NIH study in *JAMA* confirms that the benefits of quitting "outweigh" the risks. Smokers are heart healthier if they quit, even if they gain 5 to 10 pounds after quitting.

Smokers who quit before age 40 have a life span almost as long as people who never smoked, according to a Canadian research team's study in the *New England Journal of Medicine*. Smoking cuts at least 10 years off a person's life span.

Husbands may provide less effective support to women who are trying to quit smoking than wives give to husbands.

Women may be more susceptible than men to environmental cues to smoking, such as smoking with certain friends or smoking associated with specific moods. Many women may enjoy the feeling of control associated with smoking a cigarette.

Yet according to researchers at the Moffitt Cancer Center in Tampa, nearly 50 percent of pregnant women who smoke will quit during their pregnancies, but more than half of those will start smoking again after they give birth. Not only is smoking harmful for new mothers, but their babies could also be exposed to dangerous secondhand smoke or thirdhand smoke (now recognized as a danger when smoke particulates land on surfaces, in a car, for example, even if the children are not in the car while someone is smoking).

Just as men are more apt to quit "cold turkey," women, because they are from a different planet, will stop and ask for directions. Therefore, women are more likely to ask for help when trying to quit smoking, according to a national Yankelovich survey conducted for the National Women's Health Resource Center. With so many quitting options for smokers, it's critical for smokers to enlist the support of their doctors.

But is your doctor prepared to help you quit?

We're not doing enough in our medical schools to train medical students to help their patients quit smoking. Part of the problem is that we simply don't know how to teach behavior change to our up-and-coming colleagues.

Some of the leading schools are using role-playing techniques with pretend patients, according to a report in *JAMA*. But most med schools still rely on traditional lectures and handouts, and students may have as few as three hours on smoking cessation techniques—imagine, just three hours in a four-year program when 20 percent of patients they may see in their careers are suffering from smoking's ill effects on their health.

Here is the irony. Several studies have shown that smokers would quit if their doctor told them to. But when nicotine-replacement therapies, such as patches and gum, became available over-the-counter and did not require a doctor's prescription, in mid-1996, their effectiveness in helping people quit went down. Why? Because doctors were not in the loop on the counseling end anymore. Just having the doctor tell the patient to quit increases the chances of a positive outcome.

When a doctor prescribed the gum or patch, the doctor would discuss the need and the use of the product to curb cravings for nicotine. But when nicotine-replacement products were available practically everywhere, smokers were not getting the behavioral counseling component so essential to quitting. Smokers' quit lines may help replace some of the professional counseling needed to boost the effectiveness of these products.

Doctors, however, can be your best ally when you tackle this lifelong addiction. Older smokers (65-plus years of age) are more likely to quit smoking or remain nonsmoking if they see a doctor and dentist on a regular basis, according to Canadian research. Just having a regular physician and seeing a dentist regularly was a remarkable predictor of who smoked and who didn't.

In the early days of Hollywood, the movies portrayed smoking seductively: the couple enjoying a romantic, smoke-filled moment. Today, some couples who smoke together find it extremely difficult

to break that bond, despite overwhelming evidence that smoking kills. An antismoking campaign in Oregon uses a Hollywood scene to encourage quitting: He says, "Mind if I smoke?" and she replies, "Care if I die?"

Many couples, after smoking for years together, find that smoking is an integral part of their relationship, according to Michael Rohrbaugh, professor of family studies and human development and psychology, University of Arizona. When one person seeks to quit, the dynamics of the relationship can change. His research shows that family and relationship patterns contribute to continued high-risk smoking.

The ongoing challenge for research is to develop treatment programs for single-smoker couples, as well as what to do for couples who smoke when one quits.

Are you prepared to help yourself? Here are a few techniques:

- **Declare a smoke-free home,** and your chances of quitting smoking are higher. Smoke-free homes give family members an effective means of exerting social pressure on smokers living with them, and this is a powerful tool for changing the smokers' behavior, say scientists at the Cancer Prevention and Control Program at the University of California–San Diego.

- **Fight or switch?** At one time, smokers would rather fight than switch brands. But now, smokers who switch are more likely to be quitters. If smokers switch to lower-tar or lower-nicotine cigarettes for health reasons, they are more likely to quit smoking, compared with those who smoke regular cigarette brands, according to researchers. Switchers in the study of thousands of Air Force recruits, who were hoping to reduce their health risks, were less dependent on nicotine, and were more likely to have tried to quit smoking before.

- **Never quit quitting.** Often, people relapse if they smoke one cigarette or an entire pack while they're trying to quit. If this happens to you, you have not failed. The best thing to do is to try to quit again as soon as possible. After so much mental and physical preparation, such as choosing a quit date and talking with your doctor about medications that may ease the transition, it's much easier to try again soon after a relapse than to try to quit several weeks or months later. Don't put too much pressure on yourself. The first few days after you quit, you may temporarily feel tired, irritable, and develop headaches or a cough. Keep in mind you're taking the first step toward better health—even though it may not seem so at the time. Never quit quitting until you really do quit.

Smoking doesn't affect me; I don't smoke

I think we've solved the smoking-or-nonsmoking section issue in restaurants and bars, and I'm grateful for that. I don't know who we were kidding having separate sections when the entire restaurant shared a single ventilation system. Some bars have created outdoor patios for smokers.

I recommend you stay in a hotel that is completely smoke-free, not just lodgings with smoke-free rooms. Studies have shown that smoke-free rooms are never completely void of secondhand and thirdhand residue. If we can smell the smoke, it is harming us and our families.

The big issue is protecting our children from exposure to secondhand and thirdhand smoke. Children living in homes where at least one adult smokes are in danger. Being exposed increases a child's risk for developing asthma or worsening existing asthma, according to the American Academy of Allergy, Asthma, and Immunology. This group, along with the Environmental Protection Agency and other national organizations, encourages parents who smoke to do so outside their homes and cars. This goes for guests in your home and for babysitters, and should be something you consider when looking at day-care centers.

Even riding in a car in which someone has smoked, but is not actively smoking, puts kids at risk.

Tobacco smoke is more harmful to children than to adults because children's lungs still are developing. Researchers at Massachusetts General Hospital addressed parents' smoking habits when their children were admitted to the hospital for respiratory illnesses. The thinking is that the illness was caused or made worse by exposure to secondhand smoke. Many parents who were targeted in this "teachable moment" took advantage of smoking cessation programs the hospital offered.

Like canaries in coal mines, children can show the harm from passive smoking first. But for adults, by the time symptoms of lung cancer evolve, such as a nasty cough, pain, or bloody sputum (mucus from airways), most patients are beyond cure. When diagnosed with lung cancer, some smokers express regret at having smoked. But feeling guilty at that point is not constructive and wastes energy. Even with advanced cancer, it's time to stop smoking because patients who stop smoking may be more fit and better able to tolerate therapy.

Major advances have been made in the treatment of this disaster, but, generally, the final victory is not really in sight. Routine chest X-rays are not a helpful tool in diagnosis, but there is some exciting news. The spiral CT scans detect cancers when they are far smaller than those seen with a chest X-ray. The high-risk person (a pack-a-day smoker, for example) may want to check into this screening method since it has been recommended as a screening tool only for selected populations.

If you cannot stop smoking, decrease the number of cigarettes you smoke. In any given year, fewer than 3 percent of smokers quit by themselves. This is not a moral flaw or an issue of willpower. It's difficult. But talk with your doctor. Patches, medications, gum, inhalers, lozenges, and support—sometimes in combination with each other—are working.

The time is right, and the best time is now. No doubt, smoking is the most preventable cause of death and disease.

Sleep: Not Enough *Zzzzzzz*

You're heard the word *circadian* used to describe sleep cycles. Circadian is a rhythm associated with our 24-hour sleep/wake cycle, and it is set by the 24-hour trip our Earth takes to rotate once on its axis from day to night and back again.

For most of us, these rotations become regular and downright routine. But if something disrupts that routine, such as jet travel to Europe or shift work on the job, you can throw off your entire metabolism, including sleep.

The body's circadian clock is a tiny cluster of nerve cells behind your eyes. These cells send out the signals that control your natural daily rhythms.

We are a sleep-deprived society. Our generation gets less sleep than almost any other in American history. Overall, Americans are getting at least 20 percent less sleep than they did 100 years ago (TV and the Internet are causing almost half of adults to stay up later than they should), and our 24/7 society is seeing a dramatic drop in productivity because of it.

Results from major research organizations, summarized by the CDC, may be a wake-up call. Sleep loss takes a toll. Look at what lack of sleep is doing to us:

- Among adults 20 and older, 23 percent of sleep-deprived individuals have trouble concentrating on things. You don't want this person to be your bus driver or your airplane pilot.
- Another 18 percent say they have trouble remembering things. Let's hope it's not your doctor.
- Believe it or not, 11 percent say they have trouble driving, and these people are not only admitting they are sleepy while driving, *they are driving!*
- Some 8 percent say they have trouble performing their work. Do you really want this person assembling your new car? Or policing your neighborhood? Or dispensing your pills? Or monitoring the nuclear plant? Or captaining an oil tanker?
- Lack of sleep can cut learning ability by up to 40 percent. Which is why kids need sleep to do their best in school (along with a healthy breakfast).

Sleep deprivation may explain why accidents happen. There is no doubt that insomnia is a national epidemic clearly affecting worker safety and worker productivity. The errors that lead up to many catastrophes occur in the early hours of the morning when the average person's attention span is clearly limited and fatigue is probably an overriding factor.

Forty million Americans report having sleep problems, according to a survey by the National Sleep Foundation. With so many people up at night and drowsy during the day, you'd think doctors would routinely quiz patients about their sleep issues. But they don't. The same survey found that 60 percent of adults have never been asked about the quality of their sleep by their doctors. Why?

If you're having trouble sleeping, talk with your doctor. It's as simple as that. This should be a routine part of any physician encounter—even if you have to bring up the subject.

A number of Mediterranean and Latin American countries have instituted the concept of the midday siesta. From both a biological and a physiological standpoint, this makes perfectly good sense, especially during the heat of the day. However, as the world becomes increasingly digitalized, this practice is eroding, much to the detriment of body and soul.

Asleep at the wheel

Driving without proper rest can be as risky as driving drunk. Sleepy drivers are much more likely to be involved in a sleep-related crash. A sleepy driver may be your neighbor who is putting in extra hours at work, or a new parent sleep deprived because baby keeps night hours. Often, overly tired drivers report not knowing how sleepy they really are and say they don't feel sleepy before driving.

The typical drowsy driver is more likely to

- Work 60 or more hours a week
- Work 2 or more jobs
- Take medications that may cause drowsiness
- Sleep fewer than 6 hours per night, leading to sleep deprivation
- Be awake for 20 hours or longer
- Drive frequently between midnight and 6:00 a.m.

It all adds up to the risk of falling asleep behind the wheel, which has the potential for causing a serious crash. Let this be a wake-up call to every driver to pay attention to sleeping patterns, and plan not to drive while sleep deprived. Drinking coffee or Red Bull, or downing one of those tiny bottles that claim to give you a five-hour energy burst, or turning up the radio, or opening a window, all are ineffective "solutions" that simply do not keep drowsy drivers awake and alert. *Only sufficient sleep can keep us awake and alert.*

Losing sleep in your quest for rest?

Various sleep disorders can affect whether you have a good night's sleep. The composer of one of the world's best-known lullabies (hum along with me: "lullaby, and good night ...") may have suffered from a common sleep disorder known as sleep apnea. Researchers have speculated that Johannes Brahms (1833–1897) had sleep apnea, which affects as many as 5 percent of Americans. Doctors in his day, however, were unaware of the risks of the condition.

Sleep apnea causes a sudden interruption of breathing, heavy snoring, sleep deprivation, and excessive daytime sleepiness. Brahms never married, but a traveling companion said no one could sleep in the same room because of his snoring. The rather large Brahms (obesity is another risk factor for sleep apnea) was known to snooze in the afternoon in the Vienna cafés where he was a familiar sight for gawking tourists.

Fortunately, new techniques are helping many with sleep apnea get relief and a sound night's sleep (and their bed partners too). With proper medical help for sleep apnea, no one would need a lullaby—not even dear old Johannes Brahms.

Bright news about the dark days of winter

With the ever-earlier end of Daylight Saving Time in most parts of the country each spring, millions of Americans may have to deal with the darkness of shorter winter days for a longer period of time, leading to a condition called seasonal affective disorder (also known as SAD).

Our internal body clocks—that circadian clock I have mentioned—depend on light signals to tell us when to be energetic and when to sleep. That's why we tend to be more active in summer and less productive in winter. There really may be something to hibernation after all!

Getting out of bed on a dark winter morning can be tough. It's especially hard in Rochester, Minnesota. I've survived 42 winters here, so I know. But for millions of people with SAD, it's even worse. Their body clocks need a strong stimulus of light, like sunlight, to reset their circadian rhythms every day. In winter, they don't receive this strong light signal, so their internal body clocks shift and produce the wrong hormones at the wrong time of day.

As the season wears on, this imbalance can cause fatigue, exhaustion, and even depression. People with SAD may have trouble sleeping and concentrating, and may also lack energy and alertness.

Talk with your doctor about symptoms of SAD. Light treatment is often recommended, in which you might sit in front of full-spectrum light to reset that internal clock. Other strategies can often help:

- Try to keep a consistent sleep/wake cycle.
- Increase the overall light in your home, especially in the morning and evening, and stay in well-lit areas.
- Make sure evening activities include light. For example, don't watch TV in the dark.
- Be active! Physical activities decrease the effects of shifted circadian rhythms.
- Light from computers and smartphones can disrupt sleep cycles, especially when used just before bedtime.

There is a school of thought among Eastern healers that the time you wake up, if you wake up in the night, tells you what's troubling you. So, for example, if you awaken prematurely between midnight and 2:00 a.m., you're feeling anger, so they say. Waking between 2:00 a.m. and 4:00 a.m. signifies fear, and if you're up watching infomercials from 4:00 a.m. to 6:00 a.m., you're feeling sadness (or just a need to shop; okay, I made that last one up, and, frankly, I don't know how much truth there is to this theory).

But I do know this: lack of sleep for any reason—sleep apnea, shift work, depression, seasonal affective disorder, a snoring bed partner—is reason enough to talk with your doctor about what may be causing the problem and figure out how to put it to rest (and not just with medications).

No Safe Sun: Indoors or Out

One morning, I walked into the exam room where a young mother was breast-feeding her newborn. Beside her were her husband and her parents. She had been diagnosed with malignant melanoma (the deadliest form of skin cancer). She was dying. Her life was in my hands—as have been the lives of thousands patients I have seen in my career as a cancer specialist.

Later the same day, another young woman was awaiting me in a hospital bed. She too had malignant melanoma, which began as a freckle on her left thigh. Because her situation was so grave, she had moved up her wedding date. She was to be married in 10 days because a planned summer wedding (just a couple of months away) now seemed far too long to wait. As I was leaving her bedside, she held out her hand and embraced mine. "Please pray with me," she said. I did.

The young mother's cancer began with an itchy mole on her neck. Both women had tanned as teenagers so that they could look bronzed in their prom dresses. They didn't expect those strapless gowns to be part of a chain of events that would lead to their horrible diagnoses—and to me.

Here's the issue: malignant melanoma. This is one of the most deadly forms of cancer that we oncologists see. It is increasing faster than any other cancer, even faster than lung cancer and breast cancer. The real tragedy, and the real opportunity, is that malignant melanoma is completely preventable. This is a cancer caused, in large measure, by exposure to the sun.

We've all heard the message, there is no safe sun, but is anyone listening?

The American Academy of Dermatology—representing the skin doctors who first see the harmful and sometimes fatal effects of too much sun—is alarmed by the number of teenagers and young adults who continue to tan indoors and out, not to mention the number of Americans who still think there is "safe sun."

There is no such thing as a safe tan. Think about what *tanning* means. When you expose your skin to the sun, ultraviolet radiation causes a reaction in the melanocytes (these are the skin cells that produce pigment or color), and your skin turns brown (theoretically, unless you've sunburned, which is even worse). The problem is not the brown color but the ultraviolet radiation that triggers a response in your DNA. Cells may go haywire and form a melanoma or other types of skin cancer.

The sunless tanners or "tan in a bottle" products can turn your skin brown or give it a bronze glow. These products put a nontoxic, simple sugar called DHA on your skin. Proteins in your skin interact with the sugars to create a tan. Though harmless, these products perpetuate the myth that a tan is good. A tan is not good. Somehow we need to change the attitude that people look better with a tan. They don't. They look like skin cancer waiting to happen.

Consider this: We use the process of tanning to turn animal skins into leather. When you process your skin under the sun, you allow the ultraviolet radiation to break down the proteins in your skin cells. Over time, you end up with premature aging and wrinkled leathery skin. It's your "hide."

Those seemingly simple sunburns that happen to teens and younger kids on beaches and at swimming pools and lakes across the country can be tracked to serious skin cancers later in life. People who say, "I burn first, then I tan," are putting themselves at great risk.

Still, dermatologists are treating more and more fatal skin cancers in remarkably young patients. The common denominator is overexposure to the sun before the age of 18 when their skin cells are especially vulnerable to injury from the sun's rays.

More than a million people a day invest time and money (and put their health at risk) in tanning salons. The damage they receive from indoor lamps is just as dangerous as outdoor sun exposure. Most salon lights provide a significant amount of UVA and UVB radiation—and both these types of ultraviolet radiation are also found in the outdoor sun and can cause various types of damage.

Think of your skin as being 8 minutes away from the sun. Damaging ultraviolet rays travel the 93 million miles in 8 minutes to inflict their harm. Stop the rays, choose your cover, and you'll lower your lifetime risk for skin cancer. You may even prevent other problems the sun causes to unprotected skin, and I'm talking about wrinkles—a sign not only of aging but of skin damage.

The Rules to Preventing Skin Cancer Caused by Sun Exposure

Sunscreen labels have changed. You won't find *sunblock* anymore. And you won't find *waterproof* on the sunscreen labels either. The FDA has created new labeling rules.

Look for *broad-spectrum* to be protected against both UVA and UVB sun rays. Buy *SPF 30* or higher, advises the American Academy of Dermatology (AAD).

There are 17 active sunscreen ingredients approved for use in the United States. Sunscreens with inorganic ingredients, such as titanium dioxide and zinc oxide, reflect and scatter the damaging ultraviolet rays. Other organic ingredients, such as OMC or avobenzone, absorb and scatter the ultraviolet light as heat. A combination of these ingredients is often called *broad-spectrum,* and it helps get SPF factors higher. The higher the number, the more protection against sunburn, but that doesn't mean you should stay out longer in the sun. When buying your next sunscreen, read the labels just as carefully as you read food labels.

If the sunscreen is water resistant, you'll also see the designation of 40 or 80 minutes, which is the amount of time it works effectively before you need to reapply. No sunscreens were ever waterproof or sweat proof anyway. And not all new sunscreens are water resistant.

Don't buy sunscreens that contain insect repellant. The AAD says you should buy two different products. Apply the insect repellant only once. The sunscreen you'll need to apply more often.

Use plenty (a generous handful for your entire body) of broad-spectrum sunscreen, and reapply every two hours you are out in the sun. Studies show that most people apply much less sunscreen than is required to achieve the SPF (sun protection factor). More is better, in this case. If you apply less, then consider that you may not get the full SPF protection.

Apply sunscreen to dry skin 30 minutes before being in the sun so that it can be absorbed by the skin and is less likely to wash off when you perspire. Note expiration dates, because some sunscreen ingredients can degrade over time.

Don't wait until your skin begins to turn red to apply sunscreen. The damage has already begun.

Wear broad-brimmed hats and protective clothing.

Avoid outdoor activities when the sun's rays are the strongest. Follow the Shadow Rule: If your shadow is shorter than you are, the sun's damaging rays are at their strongest, and you are likely to sunburn.

Seek shade but don't depend on it. Researchers at Purdue University created models showing the benefits of tree cover. They caution that even a tight canopy of leaves and branches cannot completely block the sun's rays, nor will tree shade fully protect you from harmful sun. So much for that hammock!

Skin check

As the most common form of cancer in the United States, skin cancer will be diagnosed more than a million times this year, and one person dies of its most fatal form, melanoma, every hour.

Let's talk about the signs and symptoms that might suggest a malignant melanoma.

Finding spots on your skin that could be cancerous is as simple as looking at your skin. Unlike other cancers, you can see skin cancer. It appears on the surface of the skin. Pay attention to spots that appear and then go away, only to come back in the same place. Watch for areas that are easily irritated when you towel-dry yourself. These are tiny warning signs, so listen to them.

A mole or freckle that bleeds, itches, or changes color or texture needs to be seen by a physician. Every doctor's visit is an opportunity for a skin check—even when you're there for something else. So ask your doctor to take a look, especially in areas you cannot see easily, such as your back, back of your neck, and scalp. You must take the initiative, because primary care doctors only conduct skin exams at about 16 percent of office visits and talk to their patients about skin cancer prevention at just 2 percent of their visits, according to a study in the *Journal of General Internal Medicine*.

A new mole or freckle, whether it is colored or not, should be evaluated by a physician. Pay attention to a mole that changes in color, shape, or size. One study in the *Archives of Dermatology* noted that patients often don't realize a mole is changing or enlarging. If you're concerned about a spot, I suppose you could attempt to measure it. Better yet, get it looked at, and spare yourself the uncertainty. Some patients even snap a "selfie" on a smartphone and e-mail it to their health providers.

Ask your spouse or partner to look at your back, and if there is an irregular or darkly pigmented spot, don't ignore it. Melanoma and other skin cancers can show up in areas that have never been exposed to the sun, so don't overlook any area, including between your toes, in your scalp, and on your genitals. More than half of people with melanomas found their own cancers. Women were more likely to detect theirs than men, and wives were more likely to spot something on their husbands than vice versa, according to a study by researchers at Memorial Sloan-Kettering Cancer Center.

Physicians, however, did a good job of finding early skin cancer, especially if the patient had a family history of melanoma. Family history is important information you need to know and share with your doctors.

Winter sun: It's good for you

It's one of life's cruel ironies, but for most people, some sun is one of the best sources of vitamin D (as discussed earlier in this chapter). This important nutrient makes your bones stronger and helps prevent fractures. You need about 20 minutes of sun each day, on the areas of your body that are normally exposed (such as your face and hands), to cause the chemical reaction in your skin that produces vitamin D.

How to get the sun you need: Sunlight that comes through window glass won't cause your skin to make vitamin D. But even in the winter, you don't have to park yourself in a lawn chair in the snow to get your 20 minutes of direct sunshine. In fact, you don't need to get it all at one time. You can add up the minutes of exposure you get from such activities as walking to the end of your driveway, to the bus stop, or through the shopping mall parking lot to your car.

Unfortunately, those of us who live in Minnesota and other parts of the U.S. north of warmer states can't get enough sun during winter months anyway, because the sun's angle isn't giving us direct rays. You do need to talk with your doctor about supplementing your diet with vitamin D.

Vitamin D can be found supplemented in milk and in other foods. If you take a calcium supplement, make sure you're getting vitamin D either in the calcium pills themselves or separately through sun or food or supplements.

My Prevention Rx

We are creatures of habit. We thrive on habit (good habits, that is) and the routine of life. Results from research conducted on thousands of people over three decades show clear secrets to living a longer, healthier life.

The secret is not to be found in a tabloid headline, in a pill or potion, or in a diet plan or anywhere on the Internet. The secret is found within yourself and in what you do (and don't do) every day, day after day.

- Physical activity. Choose something you will do. Don't join a gym because of a Groupon. You won't stick with it.
- Add resistance training to maintain muscle mass. Learn stretching for flexibility.

- Eat a plant-based diet when you can. Grocery shop with a list and a plan.
- Get regular health screenings for your body and your teeth.
- Find connection in your community.
- Learn to say no, because stress will eat you alive.
- Avoid tobacco and alcohol.
- Learn to sleep at least seven hours a night (or take a midafternoon nap).
- Get out of your comfort zone, push the envelope, try something new.
- Never give up serenity to someone who attacks or offends you.
- Learn meditation and mindfulness. Reflect on your day in the mornings. Guard your "alone time."

We Americans are now living longer than ever in history. The average individual life span at the turn of the 20th century was the late 40s. A high proportion of the population can now expect to live to at least 80 years of age, and possibly far longer if these prudent guidelines are followed. The choice is up to each of us to make those years productive, creative, and meaningful, as opposed to years of decrepitude dealing with the ravages not only of age but also of severe chronic illnesses.

The choice is always there. The information is available to help guide us in appropriate directions. Cancer or heart disease or diabetes or whatever is lurking in your family tree is not a "done deal," nor is it a case of roulette, a random selection of cards or a roll of the dice. We can put ourselves behind the eight-ball, deal ourselves a lousy hand, give ourselves an unplayable lie—or position ourselves so that our remaining time can be productive, creative, and meaningful. Each of us can indeed make the world a little better than it is right now. But we have to be here to do that.

But sometimes, despite all the healthful eating and exercise and "good living," we lose our health, and the journey to regain it can often take us down paths we never wanted to travel. Cancer is not the only disease that will take us on a new uncharted path; any dreaded disease or chronic condition can turn our lives around completely.

Few diseases rival cancer for an emotional blow, but we need to acknowledge that other dreadful diseases can cut us down just when we think we are on top of our game. Illness does not respect status, fame, or wealth. Focus on the coping skills and navigational tools in the following chapters. They will help you weather the storm of disease. If we are lost in the woods, the way to survive is the same whether we're lost in a national park in California or the Everglades in Florida. Starting with the next chapter, I have drawn up your survival map.

PART THREE

Essential Steps
to Surviving Any Diagnosis

8

What Do I Have?
What Should I Do? Why?

Hope is a presence that erases the limitations
on possibilities for the future.

As a practicing medical oncologist for nearly four decades, I have had the privilege of caring for thousands of patients and their families during the darkest days of their lives—and the honor of witnessing some of their most triumphant moments.

During this time, I have made some observations about mistakes patients have made. These mistakes are predictable, and you can avoid making them. I firmly believe that you, the patient, can (and *must*) be your own best advocate. And I have made some bedside observations about how best to cope with and improve your outcome from a dreaded disease—or any disease or condition, not just cancer.

You can view your medical decisions much like you might view critical business decisions. In fact, I advise you to create a board of directors (made up of your closest family and wisest friends). If you're the patient with a potentially life-threatening condition, make yourself chairman. Appoint a cabinet of advisers (this is your medical team). But, remember, you are the one sitting at the head of that table. You're the final decision maker. You're in charge.

I hope you will use the following advice as a guide to drilling deeper into the questions people need to ask when they become patients. I urge you to work with your medical-care providers to receive the thoughtful, respectful, and learned answers and care you deserve.

Know Your Diagnosis

First, you need to know what's going on with you. That's your diagnosis. If it's a broken arm, a brain tumor, heart attack, stroke, diabetes, lupus, or any other condition or disease, minor or major, you need to know what's happening so that you can access information about the problem on your own and then recover from it. Even better, if you can see the enemy, you can fight it. So insist on seeing your X-rays, lab results, CT scans, PET scans, mammograms, bone scans, and MRIs.

Acknowledge the seriousness of your diagnosis. This involves knowing the name of the cancer under the microscope, the size and grade of the cancer, and whether or not this is viewed as a slow-growing or an aggressive process. You need to know if you have type 1 or type 2 diabetes, what kind of heart attack you have had and how much heart damage you may have sustained, or whether your stroke was caused by a blockage or bleeding. Without knowing the details about your condition, you cannot access information about the problem on your own and make informed decisions about your treatment.

Let me briefly explain the difference between grade of cancer and stage of cancer. *Grade* of cancer refers to how the cancer looks under the microscope. A grade 1 cancer is quite innocent or smoldering; whereas, a grade 4 is an angry, aggressive cancer capable of spreading. *Stage* refers to the extent of the cancer in the patient's body. For example, a stage 1 lung cancer is a local spot; whereas, a stage 4 cancer has spread to a distant site, such as the brain or liver.

My best advice is this: Bring along a family member or friend (someone from your "medical" board of directors) who can think clearly and act as your advocate by asking questions and writing down the doctors' responses. Why? Because most patients retain very little information when their circuits are overloaded from being presented with a serious diagnosis.

Be in Charge

Next, create an equal partnership between you and your primary care physician or specialist. Don't give up or just go along with medical decisions made by someone else. Ask your family and friends for support, but do not proceed with treatment just because *they* think it is the right thing to do. You are all allied against a common foe (your disease), with hopes of achieving one of three goals: a cure, quality time, or decreased symptoms.

A trusted friend or adviser can reframe or reinterpret comments of the health care provider, but no one should speak *for* you.

You and your doctor have equal responsibility for the outcome, but you, as an empowered patient (or a knowledgeable family member or friend acting on your behalf if you are unable), will make the ultimate decisions about your treatment. Gone are the days when families and doctors conspired to keep the true diagnosis of a dreaded disease from the patient in order to spare him or her the fear of the outcome.

Make certain that you get copies of letters from your specialist to give to your primary doctor. Keep your operative and pathology reports, especially if you plan to seek a second opinion. Your medical records are your property, but be aware that you may not understand all the clinical terms (medical techno-speak).

Keep in mind that you, the patient (or you as the advocate for your parent or spouse or child or friend, as appropriate), need to be appropriately assertive in treatment decisions. Speak up. Be involved. It's your life. (Or the life of someone you care about or are responsible for.)

Don't ask the doctor what he or she would do in similar circumstances. It's tempting to go along with the doctor who says, "Well, if you were my mother …" or "I'd advise my golfing buddy …" They are not you.

When my patients ask what I would do, I explain that what may be right for me may not be okay for the patient sitting in front of me under the same circumstances. Here's an example. I know the risks of chemotherapy. If the chance of benefit is low, and if side effects are high, I may not elect treatment. But some patients will grasp at any remedy, even if the odds of benefit are one in a thousand. I'd opt for quality time. Some patients, on the other hand, play the odds.

Providers need to be respectful of the patient's wishes. Some individuals will offer a toxic, unproven treatment even if the chances of benefit are less than 1 percent. This is not a choice that I would make, but I need to be respectful and supportive of my patients.

My best advice? Is it obvious by now that I want patients to be in charge?

Knowledge Is Powerful Medicine

At all times, be active and appropriately assertive. You're in a foreign environment in your new role as patient (or caregiver or trusted adviser). You don't know the language or how the game is played. But you can learn, just as you may have learned about the financial world in order to invest in the stock market or learned the ins and outs of buying and selling on eBay. Knowing the language of medicine will help you talk effectively with the medical specialists holding your (or your loved one's) future.

If the provider is using terminology that you do not understand, you have the right to interrupt and ask for clarification. I admire the parents who become experts practically overnight when their child has a devastatingly gloomy diagnosis. One couple not only became experts in a very rare respiratory condition when their daughter was diagnosed, they formed a nonprofit foundation to support research, raised funds for researchers in this neglected area, set up family and patient support groups, and even published medical papers with the few experts who truly know this life-threatening condition.

Do these nonmedical people know about this condition? Yes, more than most professionals do. Where did they learn about the condition? By reading everything they could in medical libraries and online at medical-library sites, such as PubMed, by networking with patients and their families, and by asking questions of professionals who work with this disease. Plug into like-minded support and advocacy groups, if appropriate for you.

One pertinent example that is becoming more prevalent is Alzheimer's disease and other dementias. As more baby boomers become caregivers for their aging parents or become patients themselves, they and their families can become schooled in this devastatingly "slow good-bye" by contacting the local Alzheimer's Association in person or online. Because each case is unique, and each loved one will experience a different journey with Alzheimer's, it's essential for caregiver/family members and friends to understand what's ahead. Huge decisions will be made about care, medications, and living situations.

You don't have to become a world-renowned expert, but you do need to understand a medical condition before you can make appropriate, informed decisions. Use your newfound knowledge when talking with your doctor. If you don't understand what the doctor is saying, ask for clarification and insist on an answer you can grasp.

Many of my colleagues and I are seeing an increasing proportion of patients who are bringing information downloaded from the Internet to the bedside and the clinic. Or holding iPads and laptops with bookmarked sites. On occasion, this information can produce an adversarial, confrontational environment rather than a mutually respectful consultation with an easy exchange of information.

Interestingly, in my own experience it is family members and friends who typically come to the clinic armed with online information. In general, patients may be too ill or frightened to seek out information and therefore rely on the input of friends and family. This is certainly normal and appropriate, but, ultimately, the patient is in the driver's seat and makes the decision about his or her own health and welfare.

Caution: Be careful of a well-meaning friend who dumps onto your lap a pile of questionable articles obtained from untrustworthy websites, which I have discussed earlier in this book. They're usually worthless. Be leery of the friend who offers to sell you vitamins or supplements to "cure" you, even if the friend is from your church or bridge club.

The emergence of the Internet has provided us all with access to millions of websites specifically focusing on health issues. The total number of pages on the Internet has surpassed 35 billion. (Just 10 years ago, I was astounding readers with the figure of 1 billion!) The information on the Internet can be your best ally or your worst enemy. Make it your ally, by using the information from trusted medical sources in order to make yourself the smartest patient your doctor has ever treated. [*See chapter 3 for details on medical websites.*]

Social media websites, such as Facebook and Twitter, have dramatically altered some parameters for practicing medicine. Likewise, for virtually any medical condition there is an armada of blogs where individuals post their comments and their treatments. It is not consistently possible to really understand the nuances of a patient's condition on the Internet, and the information can be profoundly dangerous and misleading.

This bears repeating: Be cautious with medical information online. Very cautious. Be wary of sites sponsored by companies hoping to sell you a product. Sadly, some of the information on the Internet is flat-out wrong, dangerous, and unreliable. Do you really think if you authorize $29.95 by credit card to *cancercures-R-US.com*, you will find what others have never found? You need to be careful. If a program sounds too good to be true, it is.

Websites in which "doctors" give specific advice can be appealing but dangerous. Check out these so-called cyber docs or alternative practitioners with an independent source. You can look up the backgrounds of medical professionals on various sites on the Internet. You're looking for medical degrees from places you've heard of to establish their credibility, not a questionable "offshore" diploma or medical degree by mail order. Anyone can get a degree from universities advertising their credentialing programs on banner ads.

Comparing your case with that of a friend, neighbor, or colleague is unwise. Patients cannot be expected to understand the subtleties and nuances of each individual's case. To compare your situation with that of a neighbor with the "same cancer" or "same stroke" or "same heart attack" can be risky and dangerous, and it can also cause lots of sleepless nights. It's like comparing legal cases or financial portfolios. Each case is unique.

The Internet is transforming civilization in general, and the practice of medicine in particular, more so than any other technology in the history of the world. It has taken the telephone approximately 100 years to connect us as a global communication family. The Internet has performed the same feat in less than 100 months. So what does this mean for the patient and the family? Let me use a primitive example of myself as an amateur financial analyst.

Because of powerful search engines and financial sites sponsored by companies, I now have access to obscure information that was previously available only to stockbrokers and financial analysts. Now let me be perfectly clear. I may not have the sophistication of some of the experts, but I can get a clear sense of market trends, prudent investment strategies, and the kinds of ideas that are completely off-base and irresponsible. In a sense, the playing field has been leveled.

The knowledge gap between me as the consumer and the financial professional has been narrowed because of the Internet. I'm able to at least know the questions to ask, and I can avoid some minefields as I pilot my financial future in a murky and uncharted arena.

However, although I may have access to financial information and financial data, I do not have financial wisdom, and that's where I need the input of the professional. So it is with the patient.

Let me weigh in further on this financial and medical analogy. My wife and I recently received information about rolling over a retirement plan from one mutual fund to another. We were happy with our portfolio until the financial adviser, who had nothing to gain from this transaction, pointed out that buried in the prospectus was the annual fee for the mutual fund. Unbeknownst to us, the annual fee was 10 times more than we were currently paying.

This is what I mean when I say that we may have information about something, but we may not necessarily have the wisdom to know how to safely proceed in regard to that information. And when it comes to your health, mistakes are far more risky than playing with your mutual funds.

Explore Your Treatment Options

Your doctor will lay out your options, but the buck stops with you. I'll say this again and again: It's your decision which path you pursue. Ask about the pros and cons of medication, surgery, diet, and further sophisticated testing. Make sure you know the goal of treatment. Decide what you are "buying" with each option or combination of options. You could be buying poor quality of life after a highly toxic treatment to live a little longer, instead of opting for peaceful quality family time. One often-overlooked option is to accept no treatment, especially for certain types of cancers.

Ask your doctor these questions to help you make your decisions:

- **Is this disease curable or controllable or confinable?** Don't accept a response of "we don't know." Doctors do know certain scenarios based on the experiences of similar groups of patients with the same type of disease. Each person's disease is different, but doctors can get in the ballpark.

- **What are my chances of getting improvement from this treatment?** If you aren't satisfied with the response, seek a second opinion from another medical center specializing in the condition you have. It's your right, and it's your future. Ask your doctor for an immediate referral. Some doctors may even sense your discomfort about the treatment plan and offer to set up a second opinion. One second opinion—no more than two—should give you enough information to make a decision. Don't waste your time waiting in airports and medical offices shopping for an opinion you like.

- **Am I eligible for any experimental treatments?** Ask if you can take part in clinical trials, but be certain to understand the differences among Phase 1 to Phase 3 trials. Phase 1 studies assess new agents. These programs are designed to find the best dose of the medication, with manageable, predictable side effects. Only rarely do patients respond to a Phase 1 trial. Phase 2 agents have some promise but rarely offer a cure. Patients participating in a Phase 2 study each have the same general diagnosis. For example, lung cancer or breast cancer or colon cancer. Phase 3 studies are final checks on whether the treatments can be expanded to a wider group of patients. The effectiveness of the newer agent is compared to a standard program.

Bottom line: Get the big picture, and then make your treatment decision.

Ask for a Second Opinion

Don't be shy. Recognize the importance of a second opinion. No single institution, and no single physician or health care provider, can have complete information about every condition. As professionals, they should not be offended if you want to seek a second opinion. This is a common practice in medicine today.

If a major medical center or university has a particular expertise in your disease, it certainly makes good sense to seek a second opinion there. The local physician will almost never be offended, and if he or she is, that is even more reason to seek another opinion. Support groups in the city where the medical center is located, or bona fide groups on the Internet, can provide names of local experts. Call on one, with your doctor's support.

But be realistic, and spend your time profitably. To fly all over the country to get 17 different opinions from a variety of medical centers is bewildering and enormously expensive—not only in terms of dollars and cents but also in terms of wasted time and energy. One or two confirmatory opinions, at the most, are more than adequate to provide some reasonable directions for treatment. Avoid the paralysis of analysis. At some point, just do it: Follow treatment recommendations—or don't.

Once you commit to a course of action, be an active patient and partner in your treatment. Keep a log or diary to help you remember what was said and recommended, and why. And have some understanding of the proposed treatment schedule. If a treatment is administered weekly at a referral center hundreds of miles from home, this may not be a workable solution for you or your family.

In summary, when you're not satisfied with your diagnosis, treatment, or progress, you'll want to get a second opinion.

Take Time to Take Your Best Shot

Any serious diagnosis is devastating and paralyzing. The very words, "You have cancer," or "Your child has muscular dystrophy," overwhelm our senses of judgment and reasoning. So take time to think about your course of action before you rush to treatment.

EDWARD T. CREAGAN, M.D.

With many conditions, the signs and symptoms may have been present for a long time, not just since yesterday. Therefore, there usually is no real urgency to rush into treatment within a day or two of diagnosis (stroke and heart attacks are exceptions where lifesaving treatment must be started within hours). Keep in mind that many treatment options cannot be reversed. For example, removal of a breast or prostate is a major life-altering event.

Have some understanding of the natural history of your disease. Ask your doctor to explain the typical track record and progression. As with most situations in life, your first shot is the best. If the first-string team is not winning, what chance does the second-string have? If the first kind of treatment does not work, the patient usually is weaker and sicker, making the success of the second treatment low. Not zero. But low.

Therefore, gather all the information and opinions, and then make informed decisions to take your best shot.

Set up your support system, and keep everyone thinking positively

Social connectedness is one of the biggest factors in explaining why some patients do better with serious illness than others do. Well-controlled studies have shown that the support of family, friends, and even pets lifts spirits emotionally/mentally and boosts immune systems physically. Families need to be supportive of the patients' decisions—no matter what those decisions are.

So my best advice is to tap into your network. Assemble your board of directors, and discuss the options for care, treatment, recovery, and rehabilitation. And remember who's chairing the meeting: *you.*

Do not second-guess your health care decisions

Don't look back. Plan ahead. Trust your instincts on your treatment, and maintain a comfort level with your care-providing team. If you don't think someone is acting in your best interest, get someone who is.

244

Let me share with you an example of a best-case scenario. One patient had early-stage breast cancer, for which the options after surgery were bewildering. Radiation, yes or no? Chemotherapy, yes or no? Hormone treatments, yes or no? The patient and her family prudently accessed responsible Internet sites. They were armed with the right questions to ask and sought two medical opinions, which basically agreed. The patient moved ahead with a sense of certainty she had made the right decision for her situation.

On Monday morning, everyone is an expert quarterback. This also applies to picking winning stocks and horses. Energies need to be focused on today and not on past events. To ruminate over diagnostic tests that should have been done or treatments that were not effective simply takes energy away from the task at hand. Focus on relationships, priorities, and the to-do list. What is important becomes obvious: family and friends, not all the other "stuff" that distracts us.

Seize the day. Savor each opportunity. After all, today is really all that any of us has.

Life Is a Full-Time Job—Set Priorities

Don't let the rest of your life unravel while you deal with treatment. Life when you're healthy is a full-time job. Be realistic when you're operating at less than 100 percent. Cut back. Slow down and smell the roses.

Recognize that there is no such thing as Superman or Superwoman. Fighting a disease, too, is a full-time job. It is foolish to think that you can deal with the rigors of certain treatments, such as chemotherapy or physical rehabilitation, maintain a business or an active work life, and run a household without some sort of help.

Nobody can go it alone, and now is the time to reach out and seek the help you need from friends and neighbors. Acknowledge the importance of a support system. A friend or confidante can be an anchor during stormy times. Don't ignore the resources of your religious group, if you have one.

Acknowledge your limitations. As a result of treatment, your energy, vitality, and focus may well diminish. It is not reasonable to continue to work 50 hours a week, reshingle the roof, and put on a dinner party for the country club crowd, all while dealing with serious side effects or recovery challenges. Prioritize, make lists, acknowledge that there are limitations to your stamina. Do not hesitate to tell people that you need rest and time alone.

Take charge of your time. If you work 60 hours a week, understand that you may not have the energy to keep up that pace during treatment and recovery, so do what's most important in the first half of your day. It's up to you to decide what's most important and how to spend your time profitably.

My best advice: Time will take on new meaning. Make the most of it.

My Survival Rx

When faced with an alarming diagnosis, many people don't know what to do, or what to do first. I've set out the essential steps to surviving any diagnosis.

Some of my patients face grim decisions about equally bleak futures. One thought that keeps me going is that hope is a presence that erases the limitations on possibilities for the future. The absence of hope eliminates any possibilities. With my patients, we never give up hope.

Whatever you face, I advise you to be appropriately optimistic, appropriately proactive, and appropriately realistic. Please recognize that there is a window of uncertainty as the journey of life unfolds.

We in medicine must embrace life's uncertainties because we don't have all the answers.

9

The Search for Health, Peace, and Serenity in Complementary Medicine

If we look too far into the future,
we miss the magic of the day.

Many people, when grasping for help with a life-threatening illness, give up on scientifically proven, mainstream medical care, believing that if they go to Greece or the Bahamas or Mexico, they will find some magic cure—usually for cancer but for other conditions as well.

I've had personal experiences where patients on this type of quest would die in a foreign hospital, thousands of miles from home. If that wasn't tragic enough, before the family could leave the local motel to rush to their loved one's bedside, the body of the deceased was stripped, rings were taken from it, and exorbitant fees were then extorted from the patient's family for the purpose of returning the body to the United States.

That's alternative medicine at its worst.

When faced with a life-threatening illness, especially one charged with a potentially fatal verdict, it is reasonable and understandable that patients will seek virtually every possible option to come to grips with their illness.

Here we are in the 21st century, with the greatest marvels in the history of medicine, the most advanced diagnostic armamentarium, the finest surgeons, and the greatest hospitals in the world. Yet there is a nagging dissatisfaction with the medical-care delivery system. An element of disillusionment exists here. Yet I can assure you there are definitely no miracle cures in Timbuktu. But I fully understand that there are patients who need to seek out that foreign country, that provider, or they will feel as if they have not examined every possibility.

What I hear every day in the clinic goes something like this: "If we can put a man on the moon, we can certainly cure cancer." But here is the problem. We have long understood the physics, the mechanics, and the engineering principles of launching a satellite to a distant galaxy. However, for most cancers right here on our planet, we do not have the foggiest notion of why one cell goes haywire, becomes bizarre, spreads, and, ultimately, takes away a person's life. Patients are frustrated, families are disillusioned, and so they seek out alternative or complementary therapies in their search for that "something else."

What's Your Alternative?

Although firm figures are not always available, many experts have suggested that at least 70 percent of patients (probably more) use techniques and interventions that do not fall under the traditional umbrella of usual and customary medical practices. I'm talking about complementary and alternative medicine, as defined by the government's National Center for Complementary and Alternative Medicine:

Alternative medical systems: Truly alternative forms of medicine would be homeopathic and naturopathic medicine, traditional Chinese medicine, and Ayurveda. Homeopathic practitioners believe that "like cures like." They administer small, highly diluted medicinal substances to cure symptoms, when the same substances at higher doses would actually cause those symptoms.

With naturopathic medicine, practitioners work with natural healing forces within the body. Such practices may include diet, massage, and acupuncture to promote healing and better health.

Traditional Chinese medicine (TCM) targets the body's life force, or qi, through diet, massage, herbs, and acupuncture.

Ayurveda, which comes to us from India, marshals the mind, body, and spirit in disease prevention and treatment.

Mind-body interventions: We'll discuss the mind-body connection further, but techniques such as patient support groups and cognitive behavioral therapy, once thought to be a little "out there," have become quite mainstream. True mind-body techniques include meditation, prayer, mental healing, and creative uses of art, music, and dance.

Biologically based therapies: Substances found in nature, such as herbs, foods, and vitamins—globally thought of as dietary supplements—fall into this category. Not everything found in nature is therapeutic, of course, and just because something is called "natural" doesn't make it safe. Lard, for example, is quite natural, but is hardly healthy.

Manipulative and body-based methods: Chiropractors manipulate muscles, joints, and tendons, and these practitioners can relieve tension and pain, but they cannot cure cancer. Many well-trained chiropractors today recognize their limitations, but they can provide relief for some people, typically working in concert with the traditional medical practitioner.

Energy therapies: Some people think that energy fields surround and penetrate the human body, although this has not been scientifically proven. Practitioners of biofield therapies, such as qi gong, Reiki, and therapeutic touch, say they manipulate the energy fields by applying pressure or manipulating the body using their hands. A more intense form of this type of therapy involves electromagnetic fields—also not proven.

These products and techniques generally are not part of the mainstream, Western medical practice in doctors' offices and hospitals. Some alternative practices have been tried and rejected, and perhaps some of those just mentioned will move more into acceptance or fall out of favor.

Let's look at past practices: At one time, there was tremendous enthusiasm for the visualization technique, in which you would sit in a quiet room and envision your immune cells gobbling up cancer cells. Unfortunately, this technique has not withstood the test of time.

Several years later, great interest was given to specific dietary regimens, such as the macrobiotic diet, which was touted as a cancer cure. Unfortunately, brown rice is not the answer.

Treatments called the Gerson Program, as well as immuno-augmentative therapy, have been popularized by a doctor in the Bahamas. These achieved great popularity but have never been proven to be of reasonable benefit. In fact, some of these practices might be unsafe because they restrict vital nutrients and certain minerals.

Some practitioners advocated enemas with coffee and other types of interventions, which are not only useless, but downright dangerous. They opened clinics outside the United States. They made considerable sums of money and offered hope with a sizable price tag. None of these treatments has ever withstood the scrutiny of appropriate clinical study.

We are now into the era of megadose vitamin supplements, and likewise these have not consistently been a benefit.

The general terminology now focuses on the concept of *complementary* rather than the word *alternative*. Complementary suggests that these are adjuncts; these are programs in addition to, rather than substituting for, traditional medicine. I don't use the term *holistic*; no one has really pinned down a definition for it.

Complementary medicine, or integrative medicine, on the other hand, combines mainstream medical therapies with alternative practices that have proven safety and effectiveness. Let me give you an example. Programs involving meditation, yoga, mindfulness, and prayerful reflection can have a very positive impact on individuals struggling with chronic pain. These types of activities can be marshaled in conjunction with traditional pain programs using codeine and morphine. Therefore, the distinction is made between *alternative* and the preferable designation of *complementary*.

It is important that your primary health care providers understand that you are participating in any type of complementary program. Research from Harvard's Center for Alternative Medical Research and Education (yes, mainstream medical schools are taking complementary medicine seriously) reveals quite a bit regarding the habits of those seeking alternative treatments.

Most people visit their primary care physician before seeing an alternative practitioner. But those seeing both types of caregivers felt equal confidence in their providers' abilities—not necessarily less confidence in modern medical practice. Most people who saw a medical doctor and used some sort of alternative practice felt the combination of the two was better than either one alone.

Among those who saw an alternative practitioner and a medical doctor, up to 72 percent did not disclose that they'd visited an alternative practitioner when talking to the medical doctor. They felt it wasn't important for the medical doctor to know, or the doctor never asked, or it was none of the doctor's business. A few felt their doctor might disapprove or discourage use of alternative medicine.

And this is where the problem lies. Sometimes serious interactions can occur between antibiotics, blood-thinning medications, and herbal remedies, for example. There's also another factor of which we need to be mindful. Patients are buying alternative medications on the Internet and at shopping malls. And we as health care providers recognize that some of these therapies either decrease the effectiveness of traditional prescriptions or enhance or accelerate side effects from traditional prescriptions.

When you buy an antibiotic or antidepressant or a heart medication at the drugstore, you can be reasonably certain that safeguards of purity and manufacturing standards have been followed. This is not always the case when you buy an over-the-counter nutritional supplement, herbal, or vitamin—even those available at the corner drugstore. So you need to be reasonable, which means sharing this information with all your health care providers—alternative and otherwise.

Worthless or Worthwhile—How Can We Tell?

The notion of complementary or alternative therapies generally refers to interventions that are not uniformly embraced by the rank and file of traditional medical practitioners. Does this mean these treatments are worthless? Certainly not. Now you're waiting for the other shoe to drop. With proper study, we can find out whether a mainstream treatment is worthwhile or worthless. And the same scientific inquiry can be used to examine alternative therapies. Here are two examples:

To C or not to C

Dr. Linus Pauling is the only person in the world to have won three Nobel Prizes. So when he spoke, the world listened. When Dr. Pauling began touting the value of high doses of vitamin C to treat cancer (he said he himself took megadoses every day), many people began adding vitamin C to their daily routines.

Many of the more skeptical medical critics said Dr. Pauling's studies were flawed. His patients who received vitamin C were compared with patient records obtained from a hospital in Scotland. This technique, called historical review, is no longer accepted as a scientific standard to assess the benefit of therapy. Needless to say, I myself was among the skeptics.

We at Mayo Clinic performed a prospective, randomized clinical trial to address this issue. The technique of our study represented the gold standard of assessing a therapy. The patients in our study had far-advanced cancer and were rigorously analyzed by a team of statisticians.

Bottom line: There was no advantage for the patients who received vitamin C in the management of advanced cancer. Our results were published in the *New England Journal of Medicine,* one of the most prestigious and rigorously reviewed medical journals in the world.

Since then, in general, high doses of vitamin C have somewhat fallen by the wayside and are no longer on the radar screen of most cancer patients.

We were strongly criticized by Dr. Pauling and his colleagues for the way we performed our study. Nevertheless, we stood our ground, and our findings (which followed rigorous scientific methods) did not show benefit for vitamin C among patients with advanced cancer.

We then performed a second study of individuals who had advanced cancer, but who also had the cancer removed surgically. For example, someone might have had a cancer arising from the colon and rectum, which spread into the liver. The cancer in the liver was removed. Though the patients were "disease-free," they were at very high risk for a recurrence of the same tumor.

These patients were generally healthier than those who had far-advanced cancer in the earlier study. We again embarked upon a trial in which patients were given either a placebo (pills with no medication in them) or a high dose of vitamin C. In the findings, once again, we could see no benefit whatsoever from the vitamin C.

Now let's take this issue one step further. Is it possible that if a person took vitamin C throughout his or her life, it would act as a preventive medication and block the development of cancer? The answers are unclear. Theoretically, maybe yes. But at the present time, there is no convincing or compelling evidence that vitamin C as a preventive intervention will avoid the development of cancer down the road. And vitamin C certainly is not without some risks.

This is the pits

Laetrile is a chemical extracted from apricot pits. It was touted as the answer to the cancer problem. A miracle cure. In the 1980s, an entire underground economy grew out of bootlegging laetrile from various parts of the world, including Mexico. These greedy "drug" dealers would do just about anything to smuggle laetrile, and cancer patients and their well-meaning family members and loved ones would also do just about anything, and pay any price, to get laetrile.

Under the direction of Charles Moertel, M.D., who had been the Chair of the Comprehensive Cancer Center at Mayo Clinic, researchers conducted a scientifically valid, meticulously detailed study and clinical trials. Again, no benefit from laetrile. And its use dropped off.

The Placebo Effect

Perhaps one explanation for the value of some of these supplements and techniques (bogus or otherwise) is the "placebo effect." In other words, if you have a strong belief that a certain intervention or a certain medication will work, it is possible that such belief will trigger the production of immune-related agents—chemicals deep within the brain that resemble opium.

This might account for the so-called "runner's high" and the ability of individuals under stress to carry on in the face of broken bones and penetrating injuries. In the medical literature there is some suggestion that about 30 percent of the benefit of a specific treatment may be related to this placebo effect.

There are a variety of brain chemicals called endorphins, which probably make us less aware of pain, and which, at least on a short-term basis, can increase stamina and a sense of well-being. In other words, if we strongly believe in the value of an intervention, it might be of some benefit, at least in the short term.

Many of us may dimly recall a history lecture that included a discussion about the mind-body connection. The first civilization to promote this concept gave birth to Socrates and Aristotle. The ancient Greeks brought many gifts into the world, and one of these was the concept that we cannot separate the mind and the body. What affects one, affects the other. Any sort of separation of these two phenomena is artificial. What we think, we become. Our language creates our reality. Attitude creates reality. If we say that today we will have a great day, guess what? We will have a great day.

Would you like a demonstration of the mind-body connection? Close your eyes and visualize a juicy lemon. See it. Feel it. Smell its freshness. Now, in your mind, cut open your lemon and squeeze the juice into a glass.

At what point did your mouth begin watering? When did your lips pucker? This wasn't a response you needed to think about. It just happened. Where did your mind end and your bodily function begin? This is the mind-body interface.

Through similar self-imagery and mindful meditative thought, you can even lower your blood pressure, calm your brain waves, and control your heart rate. Scientific studies among certain spiritual practitioners have shown that their blood pressure decreases with meditation, and there are specific changes in brain-wave function as well.

Let me tell you a story. The patient was a woman in her early 60s. She had far-advanced colon cancer with extensive involvement of the liver. The capsule of the liver is much like the covering of a football in terms of texture and thickness. It is filled with delicate nerve endings that are incredibly sensitive to the pain caused by the liver expanding from the growth of the cancer. This patient was admitted to the hospital with severe pain.

She made a clear statement to each of us on rounds one morning: "If I were a dog, you'd shoot me. If I were a horse, you would put me down. Please end this misery." We marshaled the best narcotic regimen that medicine can bring to the bedside. We brought to the patient the most sophisticated computer-driven technology to meticulously deliver doses of pain-numbing medicines. Our results were increasingly futile over the patient's first few days in the hospital.

A member of the medical team asked during a morning visit, "Do you have a church affiliation or a minister who might be of some help? What is your belief system?"

Almost miraculously, our patient's demeanor changed, and she agreed to visit with one of our chaplains. And then her story unfolded. It was a tale of betrayal, resentment, and bitterness about a devastating blow she and her husband had endured from an uncaring corporate giant. Once she found a kind listener, she could verbalize her anger at the unfairness of life. At that point, we were able to dramatically decrease the doses of morphine, and she was discharged virtually pain-free.

The lesson is clear. This is not rocket science—or even medical science. We can drip in all sorts of narcotics to relieve the patient's pain. However, we must acknowledge that many of us have pain in the soul, and if that pain is not addressed and acknowledged, it will continue to increase. This is especially true when pain in the body is simultaneously present. Consequently, it is highly unlikely that all the morphine in the world will bring such patients the peace and serenity they so desperately need.

Placebo? Or mind and body at work? Does it matter, as long as the patient finds help, hope, and healing? We need them all in our arsenal. And, equally important, we need to listen to the patient's story.

The Irony of Herbs and Vitamins

I'm supportive when patients want to try herbal remedies. I'm understanding about vitamins. But I try to point out the potential problems in taking any of these dietary supplements—they're not regulated, they could contain a host of contaminants, and so on. I try to discourage patients from wasting a lot of money and creating what some colleagues call "expensive urine" (because what your body does not use, you excrete).

Although experts say most herbs are safe when taken as directed, a recent series of FDA warnings and product recalls underscores the fact that these products are not tested, inspected, or given a seal of approval—by anybody. The Dietary Supplement Health and Education Act (DSHEA), passed in 1994, does not require manufacturers of herbs and other dietary supplements to prove that their products are safe or effective before they hit the shelves. Manufacturers can make general health claims on their labels, without any regulation about what they say.

You are unprotected when you buy herbals, In fact, a professor at Duke University Medical Center said, "You know more about what is in a bag of Doritos than what's in an herbal product touted to treat and prevent disease." It bears repeating to emphasize that there's no guarantee these products are safe or effective.

Death, liver damage, seizure, heart attack, and stroke all have occurred as a result of consumers using a small number of herbal products, according to FDA alerts and advisories. The most recent of these included ephedra (ma huang), ginger, gingko, valerian, and St. John's wort, among many others. Such adverse events can be caused by herbal products interacting with other medicines, causing allergic reactions, having impurities, or being taken in dangerously high doses.

Like many of the known risks of herbal medicines, these hazards were revealed after the products went on the market. In a sense, you are the laboratory test animal.

Still attached to your herbal of choice? Certainly hedge your bets, and don't create dangerous interactions. Be aware that herbals and prescription medications may not mix well. Discuss everything you take with your doctor. Pharmacists are also quite expert in reviewing drug-herbal interactions; in fact, pharmacists may be even more skilled than most physicians in this area.

Open Your Mouth and Say "Om"

Scientists are not quite certain how meditation works, but perhaps we can gain some insight from the work of Harvard's Herbert Benson, M.D., who initially wrote about the relaxation response. Dr. Benson's work has shown that images of a quiet stream or a flower-laden forest can lower blood pressure, lower pulse, and have tremendous benefits for those with coronary artery disease.

Picturing serenity, achieving bliss in your mind's eye—this is the very basis of human pursuits. Through mental imagery and meditation techniques, prayer, and other types of cerebral activities, people fight disease. Whether or not these techniques prolong life is unclear, but they certainly enhance the quality of life and empower patients in this most difficult of all of life's journeys.

The meditation program called mindfulness-based stress reduction has been developed for patients with chronic illnesses and conditions, such as anxiety/panic disorder, asthma and allergies, cancer, depression, gastrointestinal problems, high blood pressure, chronic pain, sleep disorders, and stress.

Researchers reporting on the mindfulness technique say that nearly all participants in the study were continuing their meditative practices a year after the initial eight-week program. The training helped these patients cope with illness and stress. They were able to learn deep-breathing techniques to reduce body tension and increase mental clarity. Overall, they simply felt better and were better able to cope with their illnesses.

Meditation techniques are not a secret. Nor are they difficult to learn. You can find worthy programs taught through wellness and fitness centers, at universities, in hospital programs, and at yoga centers.

The meditation or yoga mantra—a word or phrase that you repeat silently to trigger the relaxation response described by Dr. Benson at Harvard—can be powerful. Similar to prayer, the mantra can create measurable beneficial effects in your body. A study in Italy recorded the breathing rates of adults who either recited the rosary prayer or their yoga mantra. Both the mantra and the Ave Maria slowed breathing in the test subjects, improved their concentration, and induced a sense of calm and a feeling of well-being.

And then there is the power of prayer.

One of the first efforts to study the effects of complementary medicine practices was conducted at Duke University Medical Center, with cardiac patients who required coronary stenting (a heart procedure to prop open the arteries).

Patients who received complementary interventions, in addition to the stenting, appeared to do better than those who simply had the operation. All patients received the stenting, but smaller groups of these patients also received one of four interventions: guided imagery, stress relaxation, healing touch, or intercessory prayer (prayer groups of varying denominations around the world were given the name, age, and illness of the patient assigned to them, and then they prayed for the patients). Patients did not know whether they were being prayed for, or whether they were receiving standard therapy without the prayer intervention. (Patients involved in the other three interventions participated actively in those techniques.)

Those receiving any of the four complementary interventions had lower absolute complication rates and fewer problems after surgery during hospitalization. Researchers suggest that the interventions helped patients feel more calm, which helps in the recovery process. Those assigned to receive prayer appeared to fare even better than those receiving the other types of complementary treatments *and* better than the control group. The results of this pilot study were so intriguing that others studies were undertaken to test this idea.

A Mayo Clinic study assessed the impact of prayer in a randomized trial in which patients did not know if they were being prayed for by others. There was no obvious impact from the way the study was done. We just could not show benefit in this particular trial.

And, hold on, in 2006 Harvard's Dr. Benson and colleagues tested whether intercessory prayer itself or the knowledge that others were praying for the patient would influence outcome. It did not help.

We cannot dismiss the value of prayer. Simply because we cannot prove the value of an intervention, does not prove that it is valueless.

My personal retreat

Earlier I discussed how I go off the grid for three days, typically in April, to go to a silent retreat. The tone of the retreat follows the philosophy of St. Ignatius Loyola, the founder of the Jesuits. He believed that only with true quiet meditation and introspective reflection could one truly understand and tackle the great mysteries of life.

A Jesuit retreat master delivers two or three brief homilies throughout each day. These last no more than 10 or 15 minutes. An hour or two of reflection follows each homily. The campuslike grounds are beautiful and are conducive to trying to sort out who we are and what our purpose in life really is. Overall, there is a Catholic dimension to the program in terms of rituals, the Mass, and the rosary. Yet some in attendance are non-Catholics. We are each in the same boat. The issues with which we struggle are clearly universal and apply to each one of us.

As a compulsive note taker, I quote faithfully and write down some of the key issues. Let me share with you what I wrote down following one retreat.

- **Don't worry too much.** Scriptures tell us that if you worry too much, you may not go the distance in life, and that no one ever added an inch to his or her life by worrying. It's also not good for your heart. Sacred scriptures and writings from a variety of traditions are a great source in comforting patients and sustaining them in these difficult times. (Such writings also sustain and greatly comfort the doctors caring for such patients.)
- **Be cheerful and enthusiastic.** Now, obviously, this may not be possible if you are gravely ill, but the negative, whining person will drive away his or her cast of thousands.
- **Live in the present.** This means, don't look too far down the road. We're not encouraged to be foolhardy and not prepare for the future, but if we look too far into the future, we miss the magic of the day. This philosophy dovetails with the notion of mindfulness, where we become engaged and focused on the moment, rather than being

distracted by regrets of the past or the uncertainties of the future.

- **Be tidy.** This might sound like a funny recommendation, but if we spend most of our lives looking for things, obviously, we've wasted lots of opportunity and energy. Peggy and I felt we had lost our moorings when our home was torn apart for remodeling. Chaos is not creative.
- **Within reason, try to be peaceful. Mend fences.** To be angry and hostile, and to lash out at friends and colleagues or at the system, wastes lots of energy and is incredibly negative and counterproductive.
- **Be resourceful.** Figure out a way to make things happen. (A way that is *reasonably* within your control.)
- **Reach out to others.** No person can go it alone. But know when to seek solitude.
- **Delegate.** A comment was made about a prominent Jesuit theologian, Father John Powell. He became physically drained and spiritually exhausted; he was unable to function. Why? He viewed himself as Atlas trying to hold up the world. We need to delegate. We need help, and this is especially true if you are ill.

Mindful retreats are my alternative medicine. My personal stress relief. You don't have to go somewhere to create your own mindful retreat. A few moments of meditation—a long soak in the bathtub, a brisk walk, greeting the rising sun, sitting on the porch with a cup of tea—capture the healing power of solitude and contemplation. I recommend a healthy dose every day.

Music for the Body, Music for the Soul

Close your eyes. Now hum the theme from the movie *Jaws*. Is your heart beating faster? Do you feel fearful? Surely you pictured sharks in your mind's eye. You may not even be aware of the effect, but music can create a conditioned response. Interestingly, nuns in a convent who never saw the movie *Jaws* can listen to the same music and not picture sharks or spike a blood pressure reading.

Imagine, now, the power of music to heal.

The principle behind behavior change with music builds on the work of 17th-century Dutch physicist Christian Huygens, who discovered that clocks placed next to each other would tick in synchrony. This natural rhythm or entrainment, in which two bodies move together, becomes apparent when the beat of music prompts you to physically slow your heart rate, release muscle tension, and deepen your breath, thus producing relaxation.

Certain music—much like a meditation mantra—can calm you and help you unwind. And you can train yourself to consciously relax. Your heart rate will slow as it entrains with the rhythm of the music. Practice makes perfect, so every time you hear music that calms you (and it's different music for everyone), you can automatically trigger your relaxation response.

If you are hospitalized, think about taking an MP3 player or, if appropriate, a small bedside CD player and your favorite calming music. This may have some impact on your body's immune system and may help bring linkage and peace back to the mind-body connection.

This emerging discipline of music therapy is becoming more mainstream. Some of the more popular uses of this technique are in the hospice setting. Hospices are places where individuals may go with serious medical illnesses, although many patients have hospice care in their own homes. The life span of people in hospice settings usually is expected to be less than 24 weeks. Music has become an integral therapy to calm the mind and calm the soul during these dark hours.

A very small study in Europe looked at music in conjunction with cardiac rehab. Heart patients who were trained in aerobic exercise and listened to 30 minutes of their favorite music each day showed improvement in heart health more than a group of similar patients who just exercised. Again, a small study but a clear example of the power of the mind-body connection.

Now let's participate in the music itself. Certainly, singing is one form of vocal music therapy, but a centuries-old technique called chanting is being practiced to generate mental and physical health benefits. Chanting is akin to singing, only you repeat the "song" over and over, either out loud or silently, alone or in a group.

Chanting helps you withdraw your mental focus from worldly matters. Chanting captures sound as vibration. Vibration creates power. For example, much as high notes in song have been known to shatter crystal, chanting helps evoke the relaxation response, which is essential to meditation. Secondary benefits of chanting include regulating breathing, slowing the heart rate, evoking deeper concentration, and releasing helpful brain chemicals to elevate mood and energy levels.

Even without the meditation component of chanting, you can just chant in the shower as a way to begin a positive day, or even in the car as a way to insulate yourself from road rage during the daily commute. Experiment with special CDs recorded with chanting in various Eastern languages and using instruments such as the sitar. Practitioners say the more you do it, the better you will feel.

It would be a leap of faith to state that music therapy will make serious diseases go away, but it certainly enhances quality of life and creates a sense of well-being.

There's Something About a Wagging Tail

"I need to get home to see Max," my patient told me. I thought he was talking about his son, Max, or Maxine, his wife. But it turns out he was talking about his dog. His pet was his drive to overcome tragic illness and get out of the hospital. This encounter with a critically ill patient opened an incredible door for me—a door that led me on a marvelous healing path.

If you were stranded on a deserted island, would you want the company of your pet or your _____? (Fill in the name of the human of your choice.) More than half of people surveyed by the American Animal Hospital Association chose their pets. Think about it. Who's the first one at the front door when you come home?

We can no longer ignore the medical significance of the *bond* people have with their pets. Our pets create a balance between our minds and our bodies in the truest sense of mind-body medicine.

I suggest pets to some cancer patients to help them cope with the rigors of their disease. In fact, I consider getting a pet to be one of the easiest and most rewarding ways of living a longer, healthier life.

This same philosophy has been endorsed by the American College of Cardiology: that fur, fins, and feathers have something to do with enhancing quality of life. Obviously, we need to be reasonable. The elderly or infirm individual is hardly well-suited to care for a large animal, but under certain circumstances even a goldfish, a parakeet, or a cat can have lifesaving implications.

What is it about these creatures? A wagging tail, a soft purr, or a rub against your leg. This is unconditional love and utter devotion, and this is the only instance in which money *can* buy it. Research continues to tell us that pets, in turn, keep their owners happy, healthy, and active. My good friend Dr. Marty Becker, America's veterinarian, has documented the healing power of the animal-human bond in his book *The Healing Power of Pets*.

Marty and I have presented to audiences on the "pet prescription." Our unlikely tag team duo of cancer doctor and veterinarian is really not so incongruous. Both disciplines—medicine and veterinary medicine—can be part of the healing team. Dog and cat people will understand why the pet prescription works in amazing ways. The medical research literature bears this out, so let me highlight what we know.

When you stroke your pet, within minutes your brain releases a spa treatment of brain chemicals that makes you feel good—and your pet receives similar benefits too. "Heavy petting" creates a sensory reaction similar to what takes place when a mother nurses her baby. This type of therapeutic touch really works.

Petting pets lowers blood pressure; perhaps that's why pet owners take less medication for high blood pressure and high cholesterol. This puts pet owners at a reduced risk for heart disease. Even among people who suffered heart attacks, pet owners had a four times better chance of surviving for a year than did those who did not have pets.

Owning a pet can be a wonder drug all its own. The American Heart Association reports that pet ownership not only creates a healthier lifestyle with more physical activity and lowered stress levels, it has also been shown to lower blood pressure and cholesterol as a result, which brings new meaning to pets warming your heart.

Speaking of BFFs, another study at Miami University and Saint Louis University looked at the benefits of pet ownership. The researchers reported that pet owners fared better in terms of well-being than nonowners on measures of self-esteem, for example. Pet owners were more physically fit and outgoing.

Some people's pets can alert them to low blood sugar if they have diabetes; other pets can sense a heart attack or asthma attack coming on. These are rare animals who perform such lifesaving activities. Don't trust your feline or canine with this task, however.

If you have arthritic hands, massage your pet. You'll both feel better. People with AIDS who have pets are less likely to suffer from depression than others with AIDS who don't own pets.

If you will recall the relaxation response discussed earlier, you can achieve that state of calm with pets as well. Especially if you have chronic pain, a pet can take your focus off your pain and elevate your mood. The physical contact with pets can block transmission of pain and shut down your pain centers. High-tech imaging has actually shown reduced blood flow in pain areas when the "pet prescription" is taken as directed.

Pets keep you moving. Sometimes your best exercise partner is your dog. There's nothing like that Yorkie "look" or a nudge from a Labrador retriever's nose to get you off the couch and onto the sidewalk. Pet ownership, especially of dogs, gets you outside and into more social interactions. And you will recall the social connectedness theme I have been advocating. Walk your canine, and you'll meet your neighbors.

Like a K-9-1-1, pets can buffer your reaction to acute stress, as well as diminish perceptions of stress. A few minutes alone with your cat or dog might do more to help your stress than talking about your troubles with a best (human) friend or spouse.

Therapy animals, mostly dogs, are commonplace in hospitals and nursing homes. Why? Because they bring something we doctors can't find in pills. Medical-care centers are bringing in animal-assisted therapy teams—usually certified dogs and their well-trained humans—to go from room to room, bed to bed, with their own gentle brand of just "being there" for patients. We at Mayo Clinic had the wonderful opportunity of publishing a magnificent book about Dr. Jack, the helping dog. Therapy dogs change our lives. Dr. Jack was an actual member of the Mayo staff (and had his photo in the staff directory) until his retirement in 2013.

Pets bring measurable joy to people in long-term care facilities too. Animal-assisted therapy effectively reduced the loneliness of residents who wished to receive the therapy. Many nursing-home residents have had a strong life history of relationships with pets as an intimate part of their support system. Perhaps that's why nurses have observed residents with dementia who had not spoken to daughters or sons or grandchildren talking animatedly with therapy golden retrievers.

If given the choice (and many of the elderly cannot have pets where they live, which should be a defining factor when you seek a care facility for your loved ones), the elderly would choose to continue that pet bond.

Older people with pets do much better in warding off depression. They're better able to withstand social isolation. Having a pet helps them be more active. Lest you think that's because they take dogs for walks, cat owners showed an equally higher rate of life-enhancing activity. And I haven't seen many cats on walks lately.

On the other end of the age spectrum, children undergoing dental or medical procedures will feel less pain when a dog is present—and not just at their side. Kids said procedures were less painful even when the dog was curled up in the corner of the exam room.

It's not just a dog-and-cat world. People with physical, psychological, cognitive, social, and behavioral problems, such as cerebral palsy, developmental disabilities, and depression, even chronic abuse and eating disorders, are learning the healing power of riding horses. (This is known as hippotherapy, but it has nothing to do with hippopotamuses.)

I've known many people whose health went rapidly downhill after their pet died. Marty tells me veterinarians have observed this same pattern. Often, a beloved pet might be the most significant factor in motivating a seriously ill person to stay alive.

For my patients, I make a note in their medical records of their pets' names. And when the patient returns to see me, I ask, "How's Reggie?" or "How's Boots?" I find that this really eases some patients' anxiety about coming back for treatment.

Pets have a positive influence on our health because we all need something to live for and something to focus on besides ourselves. Self-absorption is terrible for your health. Pets accept us, no matter what. This unconditional love is even better, say some research studies, than admiration of friends.

I think part of the reason we connect so strongly with animals in general, not just pets, may be their emotional depth. Elephants mourn, even cry. Non-pet owners are, by now, shaking their heads. But who can question the unselfish love a pet has for you? Pets depend on us. Family may not. And we all know it feels good to be needed.

Best medicine money can buy

Let me share with you a powerful story about the depth of the animal-human bond. Several years ago, I received a phone call from a close family member who is one of the most accomplished anesthesiologists at a major medical center. His specialty is cardiovascular anesthesia. He is responsible for the life-and-death decisions of patients receiving heart transplants. This is emotionally draining and physically demanding work. Some of these surgeries take 18 to 20 hours.

When he called me, he was obviously shaken. I could hear his distress. He was inconsolable, and the sobs were palpable through the phone. My initial thought was that a family member had died or there had been some catastrophe at work. Not so. His beloved golden retriever, Sadie, had to be put to sleep. Sadie was a part of the household, a true member of the family. Sadie began losing weight and was taken to the veterinarian. The veterinarian suspected some minor liver ailment and advised an exploratory procedure.

With the beloved animal sedated, the veterinarian was horrified to note that much of the abdominal cavity and the liver had been replaced by a highly virulent malignant tumor. All agreed that the best thing was to give Sadie the easy way out by euthanizing her.

This was one of the most painful decisions of his life. A man who held others' lives in his own hands every day was completely torn apart over the loss of his family dog.

This was my own experience with Molly, and perhaps you have had these defining moments as well. Molly was our beloved Lhasa apso. A 10-pound creature who brought joy to our hearts. Then the ultimate irony struck. Molly developed malignant melanoma on the floor of the tongue, with extensive involvement of the lungs, liver, and brain. I will never forget the day that we brought her to the vet for her final trip. Her sad brown eyes looked up at us, basically saying, "It is okay. You did your best. You gave me your best shot, and I now know what needs to be done."

We agonized over this decision for weeks before that final journey. Molly's labored breathing, obvious pain, and physical deterioration were clear signs that the end was in sight. Animals become part of our souls, and animals can take a piece of our soul, but that is simply the way life is. Animals can soothe our souls as well.

And now enter Brinkley.

A week or so before Christmas some years ago, Peggy and I were called to see a little puppy at the animal shelter and to consider adopting him. It was a frigid December day with waist-deep snow. We trudged up the walk, and our lives were changed forever.

He was called Chance by the people at the shelter because that indeed was what his life was all about—another chance. One of a litter of golden retrievers, some accident had befallen him. His rear right leg was so badly injured, it had been amputated.

These big brown eyes—eyes of forgiveness, eyes of peace, eyes of compassion—looked up at us. Bingo, out came the checkbook, and things were never quite the same.

This little creature, to whom life had been unfair, now offered us unconditional love, unconditional acceptance, and unconditional forgiveness. He became somewhat of a TV star, having appeared on a local television station, and also became one of the stars of the

Mayo Clinic website after his picture accompanying our story on the healing power of puppy love proved amazingly popular.

Now where did the name Brinkley come from? For some reason, the name Chance did not fit this little character, but if you've seen the charming movie *You've Got Mail*, you'll remember the final scene in which there is a beautiful golden retriever named Brinkley. We were struck by this scene.

Our star recently left us with broken hearts. He had more pressing business somewhere in doggy heaven providing bedside therapy for others.

The take-home message: While we may have saved Brinkley's life, he really saved ours. He gave us some of the best medicine money can buy.

Not a Laughing Matter

Can you find healing on Netflix? I think so.

Norman Cousins, longtime editor of the *Saturday Review* and faculty member at a medical school in California, wrote a fascinating book called *Anatomy of an Illness as Perceived by the Patient: Reflections on Healing and Regeneration*. Cousins was diagnosed with a severe type of arthritis involving his spine. This condition is called ankylosing spondylitis.

My sense is that Cousins was given a fairly grim prognosis. He realized in his own life the tremendous value of laughter in putting a more positive spin on a desperate situation. He spent many hours watching movies with the Three Stooges and roared with the enthusiasm of an adolescent at some of the antics of Larry, Curly and Moe. Cousins indicated that his recovery was related, at least in part, to his ability to simply let go of the situation and let it unfold.

Now why should humor be such a powerful tool? It is clear that certain molecules or brain chemicals (endorphins), secreted from deep within the brain, trigger the placebo effect. These types of molecules achieve a high blood level during times of stress, such as running a marathon (the "runner's high") or when involved in an automobile accident. These hormones provide a feeling of wellness and euphoria, and may have something to do with augmenting the immune system.

Should a comedian be part of the medical team? Obviously, that would not be appropriate. However, emerging studies from social science and psychology tell us a sense of lightheartedness not only acknowledges the futility of life but also underscores the humanity of the caregiver. Humor also acknowledges that in a real sense we are all patients. We are simply at different points along the journey.

Patch Adams is a fascinating West Virginia physician who recognizes the incredible healing power of humor. He embraces the relative futility of what medicine can offer some patients. He does this through humor, with its infinite healing power. Watch the movie *Patch Adams,* and you'll see what I mean.

My Serenity Rx

A hunger in the soul of every patient is a bond or a connectedness with the physician. The physician who recognizes the humanity of the patient, and of himself or herself, has a unique gift to bring to the bedside.

As the doctor and the patient and family become more comfortable and get to know each other, a bizarre and wonderful bond forms. For me, this is quite unlike the attachment in any other medical specialty because of the emotional impact of the type of medicine I specialize in. There are incredibly rich moments of lightheartedness that patients share with us during these tender times. All of a sudden, smartphones and digital tablets fade by the wayside. Patients focus on each day as it arises and are able to see some of the absurdity in life.

A middle-aged farmer was dying from an advanced cancer. Prior to his illness he had been negotiating with a roofing contractor to replace the shingles on his farm home. The contractor he had finally selected offered him a 50-year guarantee that not one shingle would ever need to be replaced. With a wry sense of humor, this patient finished the story, "Heck, Doc, I don't even have 50 days left, let alone 50 years, but I got a good deal on the shingles."

And another touching story. I was caring for a wonderful woman who was succumbing to advanced breast cancer. Her devoted husband was at her side during the revisit. It became clear that the cancer was progressing; our options were limited.

With a sly smile, the patient asked me, "Doc, how long do I have?" I asked the patient why this question was important to her, and here is what I heard: "Since my time is limited, I want to max out his credit cards so there's nothing left for the second wife." Knowing their devotedness to each other, we all had a hearty laugh during a difficult time.

We are all patients. We are simply at different points on the journey. We physicians can certainly understand the need of patients to seek alternative practitioners. But I urge you to be realistic in your search for health, peace, and serenity.

10

Attitude Matters: The Psychology of Survival and Longevity

*Each of us has the gifts and skills
to make the world a little kinder, a little softer,
a little better than it is right now.*

Almost every day in the clinic, I see patients who do not conform to what is described in medical textbooks. What I am trying to say is that these people had dreadful prognoses, based upon a pathology report, a CT scan, a PET scan, or what we observed in the operating room, yet they have continued to do amazingly well.

We sample blood and look for patterns in their immunology. We perform a variety of tests on their hormones. But there does not seem to be a consistent theme from what we can see in the laboratory studies. Of course not. The answer to their success lies elsewhere. Each of these patients does seem to have several traits in common.

Bottom Line: You Can Survive Just About Any Diagnosis

When I reviewed much of the world's medical literature on the subject of survival, three themes emerged with long-term survivors:

- **A sense of religion.** By this, I mean individuals participating in the set of rules and regulations for certain belief systems, faith-based in many cases, but not necessarily.

- **A sense of spirituality.** Many definitions exist for this term, but the one that works for many of us is the questioning of the ultimate purpose of life: Why are we here? What is this all about? It is an attempt to find meaning, purpose, and cohesion in a sea of chaos and confusion.
- **A sense of connectedness.** You know them. They are your parents, neighbors, coworkers, and, I hope, you. These people typically have long-term meaningful adult relationships with spouses or partners, or are members of a community that gives them support and encouragement during times of crisis. The isolated individual, the disenfranchised "grumpy old man," generally does not do well when faced with adversity, and few people want to be around him or her.

What Can We Learn
from the Long-Term Survivor?

While having the privilege of being the attending physician on the Oncology Service at one of our hospitals, I have had a number of experiences that have brought home some solid, time-honored truths.

Let me set the scene. The oncology ward consists of about 25 to 30 patients, most of whom have far-advanced malignant disease. Some of them were admitted to the hospital for the evaluation and management of complications related to their cancer treatments, which include nausea, vomiting, pain, and related miseries.

Fortunately, with aggressive management many of these symptoms can be controlled so the patients can spend their remaining time in relative comfort and dignity. As I make rounds in the hospital and visit with these patients and their families, several observations are noteworthy:

- On the nightstand next to the patient's hospital bed, I do not see stock portfolios, certificates of achievement, or an acknowledgment of having been a good and faithful corporate soldier. What I do see are snapshots of children, grandchildren, and pets, wedding photos, and religious mementos, such as Bibles, rosaries, and related accessories.

- The discussions I have with these patients never focus on accomplishments, achievements, or wealth. Discussions almost always focus on missed opportunities, remorse, regrets, and "what I would have done if I had more time."
- What I hear from many patients and their families is the ache in their souls concerning what might have been, how good they could have been, how differently life might have unfolded, and how they should spend their remaining time.
- We each need programs, projects, and proposals to get us out of bed on a Monday morning. When faced with life-ending illness, the paycheck becomes irrelevant. We need to contribute, we need to feel part of a greater good, and, finally, we need to remember that each of us has the gifts and skills to make the world a little kinder, a little softer, a little better than it is right now.

Who are these patients—these heroes of everyday life? We see them everywhere. These are the anonymous faces of simple citizens who somehow continue to thrive in the face of life's unfairness, who continue to somehow dodge the bullets fired from the barrels of poverty, alcohol, abusive relationships, and just plain bad luck.

- The young single mom working the swing shift in a factory
- The midlife homemaker suffering in silence from the anguish of divorce and a bitter custody battle
- The seasoned executive banished by an MBA younger than his son to a professional gulag where the only exits are a gold watch (actually gold-plated), a heart attack, or a forced early retirement

Yet, somehow, people like these continue to suit up every day, tough it out, and have productive and meaningful lives. Now add a serious, life-threatening illness or injury. Does everything stop? Or do they march on, suit up, and give it their best shot?

What can we learn from the long-term survivor of a dreaded disease or serious injury or accident?

A lot. The hacking cough that doesn't quite go away; that vague indigestion accompanied by weight loss; a heart attack; a stroke; the brain injury that causes coma; the painless lump—each can be the start of a journey of terror and fear. Every patient's nightmare: "I'm sorry to tell you that you have cancer." "Your father has suffered a stroke; he will have a long road to rehabilitation and may never regain his ability to talk." "You have multiple sclerosis." "Your son has had a serious car accident and injured his brain." At one time, such pronouncements clearly signaled the end of the road for many patients.

But not today.

Patients are living longer than ever before with diseases and injuries that would have brought premature death to their parents or grandparents just a few decades ago. The proportion of long-term cures and medical marvels continues to increase, and for the patient who cannot be cured, there have been major advances in managing the symptoms and complications of the disease and also the treatment.

A tale of two patients

The date: December 12. The place: Room 4162 on the cancer unit. Two patients in adjoining beds have identical diagnoses. Each has advanced cancer of the pancreas, which has spread into the liver. Cancer of the pancreas is one of the most virulent and aggressive cancers. The average survival is limited to a few short months in those circumstances.

Each patient was told about the need for recovery following surgery, and a follow-up appointment was made for a month after dismissal from the hospital. One patient returned looking miraculously well, even though the cancer had slightly progressed. On the other hand, the other patient had markedly deteriorated, with profound weakness, weight loss, and an unraveling quality of life.

What was the difference in the course of these two patients? This is the sort of question that makes medicine fascinating.

I asked the obviously well patient what he did to try to keep this monster under control. Here was his game plan. When he left the hospital, he posed the following questions and challenge to his health care providers: "What can I do as a patient? What can my family do to give me the best odds of squeezing out a few extra months from this cancer? I want to participate. I want to be in charge. I do not simply want to sit back and take advice."

With this attitude, the patient sought the guidance of a physical therapist concerning an appropriate and aggressive program of stretching, reasonable exercise, and walking. He sought the input of a registered dietitian on some dos and don'ts and general guidelines about nutrition.

He made a list of what was really important for him now that the clock was ticking. He jettisoned some community committee responsibilities. He gracefully exited from commitments at work. He focused only on the one or two functions that were important to him, such as the Rotary Club and his weekly poker game.

He informed himself about the anticipated natural history of his illness, and he clearly understood the limitations and possible side effects of treatment.

Now what about the patient who was struggling for survival? What did he do? This patient did none of the above. He had a stoic, "Western frontier" mentality and thought he could go it alone, much like the Lone Ranger—minus Tonto. He became isolated from his family and friends. He did not have a list of priorities. He simply accepted what he heard about his diagnosis.

We need to be realistic. It is not possible to wish away advanced disease with happy thoughts. Nor is it reasonable to buy a lottery ticket instead of planning for retirement. But you can focus your energy on the psychological, spiritual, and social dimension of life so that you can gently shift the odds in your favor to squeeze out a few more quality weeks or months from a serious illness.

Among Jewish men there is a decrease in death rates just before the High Holidays in the autumn, followed by an expected increase just after these celebrations. Why? Perhaps some seriously ill patients have a surge of life-enhancing hormones, or are urged to eat and drink, and these could be factors. The same findings have been observed among Asian women during the Feast of the Harvest Moon.

Keys to the kingdom

When embroiled in the dark days of World War II, Winston Churchill rallied the British people with inspiring words, none so apropos for our discussion as these: "Never give in, never give in, never, never, never, never ..."

Churchill galvanized the spirit and the energies of the Brits, helping to sustain them in their valiant battle against Nazi Germany. This sort of philosophy has been used by many a coach as a team dismally fell behind at halftime. Sometimes it worked, but most of the time, I suspect, these sorts of speeches have little impact in an athletic contest. Now, let's turn our focus to an interesting medical situation.

At the present time in the war against cancer, it is appropriate and fashionable to offer groups of patients a certain treatment, let's say immunotherapy, to determine the benefit of the treatment among those individuals. In general, we hope to see benefit in approximately 20 percent of patients. When that occurs, there is encouragement to open that treatment to far greater numbers of patients. This is called a clinical trial. The assessment of an anticancer treatment among hundreds of patients gives us a good "feel" for the ultimate value of that treatment. However, the flip side of that coin sometimes is not appreciated. Not every patient will be helped. These brave souls go into clinical trials with great expectations and hopes.

It is my recollection that almost every great advance in medicine or surgery was generated by the observation of one physician dealing with one patient. The curiosity of that individual fueled additional studies and helped pave the way for some important advances. Penicillin is a case in point. Sir Alexander Fleming happened to drop some moldy bread into a dish of bacteria. Lo and behold, the bacteria were killed. Penicillin was discovered. These sorts of observations make history.

Now let me tell you about an interesting fellow. The patient was a gentleman in his mid-40s who went in for a routine examination. He was feeling generally well. To the dismay of his examining physician, there was a mass in the rectal area. A biopsy confirmed it was malignant melanoma.

The patient underwent a CT scan of the abdomen. There were extensive tumors in the liver and in the chain of lymph nodes surrounding the aorta. Under most circumstances, this would be viewed as a hopeless, dismal problem. The patient and his enormously supportive wife decided to receive investigational chemotherapy in a clinical trial. It had no benefit. He was not in the small group of patients to receive benefit from the drug being tested.

As the disease relentlessly progressed, the patient was willing to proceed with "off-the-shelf" chemotherapy, which traditionally had virtually no chance of helping. The treatment was offered during one summer, and the patient was not expected to survive. Well, that was our expectation.

Much to our amazement, shortly after the Vikings victory in the NFL playoffs, the patient called for an appointment! We were amazed and gratified that he was still with us. The patient and his wife suggested additional scans, and we discovered that the cancer was in remission. It was still present but had not spread. His physical examination also confirmed that there was little obvious evidence of cancer.

Now, what do we make of this observation? Is it a miracle? Is it simply a roll of the dice? Does it have something to do with the alignment of the planets? Obviously, any or all or none of these explanations may be adequate, but this gentleman does have some of the characteristics of long term cancer survivors—a sense of connectedness with his devoted wife, a reason for living.

So far, we do not have a brain-wave test for survival. Nor can we perform an MRI of the mind (the brain, yes; the mind, no) or devise a psychiatric profile that can predict "up front" which people will do well. But I do think that, when faced with a serious problem, the words of Winston Churchill ("Never give up") are reasonable to consider. We must embrace the harsh reality that these types of exceptional stories are most unusual, but at some point in history, these patients may provide the keys to the kingdom to help us really understand why some people do better than others.

A review published in the *British Medical Journal* analyzed 26 studies on the effective psychological coping styles and survival from cancer or its reoccurrence. The authors found little convincing evidence that attitude and disposition play a role in surviving malignant disease.

Contrary to this review, it has been my clinical experience and that of many colleagues that **we cannot discount or cast aside the relationship between the mind and the body**. I cannot dismiss my own review of the research on long-term cancer survivors (and, for that matter, it could be survivors of any other life-threatening illness) plus research showing that pessimists have a 19 percent shorter life span than optimists.

So what does this all mean? It means that we in traditional medicine do not have all the answers, and it also means that a portfolio of coping skills, including a sense of spirituality and a sense of community and connectedness, must be part of a comprehensive disease treatment program to give patients the best chance of beating the odds.

Traditionally, medicine and religion were bonded to each other. During the Dark Ages, most physicians were members of the clergy. By the Middle Ages, the church still had the ultimate authority over medical practices and awarded "licenses" to practice medicine.

One of the driving forces of this relationship was the obvious lack of understanding of physiology and biology. By the 19th century, a mechanical-biomedical model emerged as a result of advances in pathophysiology. This led to a period of so-called enlightenment in which medical illness did not reflect punishment or moral inadequacy. Attempts were made to explain virtually all human sickness on the basis of a biochemical or pathophysiologic mechanism.

In other words, individuals who contracted tuberculosis died of that infection. Individuals who had a heart attack and had blocked coronary arteries died from their illness. However, we now understand that not all patients with tuberculosis die and not all patients with heart attacks die, so there must be some other emotional and psychological factors to help explain this finding.

This old notion of illness of the body did not consider the profound importance of emotional, spiritual, and psychosocial factors affecting human illness. The medical community now recognizes that the vast majority of patients have disorders that are clearly related to emotional issues rather than to physical disease.

This fundamental concept was articulated in 1931 by Dr. William J. Mayo, who wrote: "The failure [of the medical profession] lies in an [in] ability to appreciate and deal intelligently with the emotional instabilities of those physically ill … which lead to miseries as grievous as though they were dependent on tangible physical causes."

Thus we ask the question: What is the influence of emotional and spiritual elements on disease?

My Ten Commandments for Surviving Your Diagnosis

1. **Be optimistic within reason.** See the glass as half full not half empty. Optimists do better coping with illness than pessimists do.
2. **Be knowledgeable.** Research your medical condition on credible websites and have some understanding of the natural history of your situation.
3. **Be respectful.** Acknowledge that medicine is an art and a science. There is little to be gained by being confrontational with your health care providers. We are all dealing with a common goal: the welfare of the patient.
4. **Cultivate your support system.** A nurturing support system of friends and family will honor your wishes, not their own. Keep these people close. Lose the rest.
5. **Embrace each moment.** Stay in the day rather than pontificating over the future that may never arrive.
6. **Be well.** Be mindful of your blood pressure, weight, cholesterol, physical activity level, and other wellness factors, even in the face of a dreaded disease.
7. **Understand your medications.** Know the dose, the schedule, and why you are taking every medication.
8. **Keep the team informed.** Every doctor you see for any concern needs to know your medical condition. Multiple

physicians in many offices can be a recipe for a disaster unless you keep everyone up to date on your condition.

9. **Keep copies of your medical records.** Put your wishes in writing. Have a discussion about advance directives/living wills. Appoint a health care proxy (or surrogate) to speak for you (when you can't) about your care, and make sure everyone who needs to know this information has a copy of the documents.

10. **Be appropriately spiritual.** Successful patients often undertake an inner search for meaning and purpose in the face of chaos and confusion. They find an anchor for peace and serenity during troubled times.

Mind-Body-Spirit Connection

We oncologists have at our command the most spectacular advances in immunology, imaging, and therapy for cancer. Yet we feel a nagging uneasiness that something is missing in our healing quiver. A flood of books called our attention to the mind-body-spirit connection. This literature discussed how the gravely ill patient can harness this concept to enhance quality of life and perhaps even survival.

During the mid-1980s, Bernie Siegel's book *Love, Medicine, and Miracles: Lessons Learned About Self-Healing from a Surgeon's Experience with Exceptional Patients* appeared in hospital rooms throughout the United States. This was an important work because it discussed patient involvement in dealing with cancer. He championed a heightened sense of responsibility. He encouraged patients to be active participants in treatment decisions. Patients were appropriately invited to challenge the medical institution itself and were advised not to be passive participants swept away by the armada of medical technology.

Eventually, this positive message became distorted. Some authors suggested that the "fighters"—patients who tenaciously engaged their doctors in alternative practices—and the "optimists" would somehow be granted a reprieve from their illness.

This misguided philosophy placed a dreadful burden on the shoulders of each patient. I saw this among my cancer patients, and I suspect it holds true for specialists in other medical fields as well.

Simply, the faulty message was this: Because you are responsible for your health and wellness, and because attitude is important in your well-being, if your cancer progresses or if treatment is ineffective, this clearly means you are not trying hard enough. Somehow, it's your fault if the cancer progresses. **This is simply not true.**

A more recent book, Larry Dossey's *Meaning & Medicine: Lessons from a Doctor's Tales of Breakthrough and Healing,* underscores the importance of thoughts, emotions, and meaning in health and illness, especially about cancer. Dr. Dossey's message here is that what a patient thinks has an important effect on well-being. In other words, a cause and effect. And chapters with such titles as "The Power of Belief," "Healing at a Distance," and "The Invisible Power Within" posed interesting medical questions that cannot be answered by our current methods of scientific inquiry.

In the pages of Dr. Dossey's book and other books, patients offer personal testimonials, and medical practitioners tell about their observations among patients—somehow implying that attitude and disposition can bring about physical cures and miracles. Again, the burden of responsibility rests squarely with the patients, and I see that as a dangerous idea.

We can thank these books for one thing. They created a sensitivity and awareness about the fact that patients have a responsibility to be active partners with their caregivers. But by placing the responsibility for wellness on the patients and ignoring the fact that cancer and other diseases are also a biological process—and patients don't have control over that—these books are creating a dark downside.

Where's the scientific proof?

More recently, authors of similar books are relying less on stories from single patients and are performing credible research to document the value of the mind-body-spirit connection objectively. In fact, Caryle Hirshberg, the author of *Remarkable Recovery: What*

Extraordinary Healings Tell Us About Getting Well and Staying Well, posed these questions:

- When faced with a life-altering disease, can you do anything to modify the natural history of that event?
- Can you change any behaviors to enhance quality and possibly length of life?

The authors talked to long-term survivors in an attempt to pinpoint the characteristics of these remarkable people, thereby discovering some common threads:

- Long-term survivors seemed to reach a spiritual dimension through prayer or meditation.
- Long-term survivors held an innate belief that somehow the situation would be all right.
- Long-term survivors were connected either to a spouse or life partner or to a community. In fact, some had long-term marriages lasting more than 30 years.

Now these characteristics are not a blueprint or a guarantee for survival, but they suggest that long-term survivors are not simply "lucky people" either. It also says to me that some factors influencing the outcome of cancer or other life-threatening illness can be modified.

Marriage, it turns out, is good for the heart. Married heart patients who had undergone coronary bypass surgery were more than 3 times as likely to be alive 15 years later as their unmarried counterparts, according to a study at the University of Rochester. There's something about a supportive relationship.

So what does this mean? It means that some patients with dreadful conditions do amazingly well. We do not yet have the specific probes of their personalities, but we do know that social isolation is a significant factor in mortality, and study after study shows that individuals with a sense of community and connectedness do better than individuals who are marginalized, disenfranchised, and isolated.

We must remember that although biology is destiny, we can tinker with some things in life to enhance the quality of life. We can rearrange the cards we are dealt to shift the odds in our favor.

Connectedness:
The Importance of Social Support

Let's look harder at what it means to have connectedness in life. David Spiegel, M.D., Stanford psychiatrist and author of *Living Beyond Limits: New Hope and Help for Facing Life-Threatening Illness*, divided a group of women with far-advanced breast cancer into two sections: Half met weekly and participated in a support group. The other half were not in a support group. The findings were striking.

The women who had the weekly support did far better, in terms of survival, than the individuals who were by themselves. This was an intriguing study but was viewed with some skepticism. There were some statistical flaws in the trial well acknowledged by Dr. Spiegel, and a confirmatory study has never been published, so the jury is still out on the value of support groups in prolonging survival from cancer. But there is no question that under proper circumstances these support groups empower patients and enhance quality of life.

I commonly ask some of these remarkable patients the reason for their striking survival in the face of impossible odds. The responses of these patients are predictable. First, there is a laugh of embarrassment and awkwardness. Second, patients typically use a joke or sarcasm: "Oh, I don't know. I guess I am too mean and too nasty to leave this earth."

But then they share with me the rest of the story. In almost every circumstance, it is a relationship, a person, or a pet that motivates the patient to push on and trudge forward in the face of impossible odds. A newly born grandchild, a horse that is now part of the family stable, or a renewed relationship with a long-lost sibling are the kinds of stories that we hear over and over again.

Interestingly, none of these patients has been driven by the need to increase his or her portfolio, magnify the 401(k) plan, or enhance net worth. Things and trinkets are irrelevant. Relationships and connectedness were common threads in the lives of each of these individuals.

Now is this a scientific study? Of course not, but we need to recognize that almost every advance in medicine has been made by the observation of a curious clinician visiting with a remarkable patient, and then questioning, wondering, and looking for truth—the scientific truth of why *that* patient had such extraordinary results.

I'm not surprised by the power of connectedness. Friends may be able to persuade patients with illness to eat right, exercise regularly, and listen to their doctors' advice. And while others have championed the fighter and the optimist as being best-suited to deal with cancer, it may be that these people simply have a social support system to buffer them against stress and to help them cope with their medical care. Their attitudes may have nothing to do with their illness and everything to do with seeking friends to support them during difficult times.

I am an adviser to an effective program called A Time to Heal (*mytimetoheal.org*). The two remarkable women who developed the 12-week rehabilitation program for cancer survivors saw a need. They reasoned: People who have a heart attack get cardiac rehab. Why can't cancer patients have a form of rehab after their surgery, chemo, radiation, or other treatments? Once the medical system has finished treatment, cancer patients, they discovered, felt alienated.

Drs. Stephanie Koraleski (a cancer psychotherapist) and Kay Ryan (a nurse and cancer survivor herself) convened weekly sessions for cancer survivors on such topics as spirituality, nutrition, resilience, fear of the cancer returning, the physiological aspects of cancer, medications and supplements, sexuality, relationships, and gentle exercise. For the past five years, in group after group, the findings are statistically clear from evaluations before and after the sessions: participants are happier with their lives, rate their quality of life as much better, and find connectedness within the group.

Although these sessions were intended to be informational meetings, not support groups, the 15 to 20 participants in the groups remain close with and supportive of each other and often continue to meet informally after the 12 weeks have concluded. The program has widened and spread to several cities and states.

This is just one innovative program that tapped into what psychologists have known all along about the connectedness of the human spirit in time of need.

The debate continues

Social scientists have long recognized that we have survived as a species because of our ability to band together in small clans and colonies to fight enemies, to keep ourselves warm and dry, and to feed our young. Studies of entire populations consistently make some rather interesting observations:

- People who lack social relationships are at higher risk of death.
- Being married is a plus for your health.
- Losing a spouse through death is not good for your health, especially for men.

The specific reasons why social relationships make a difference in whether you have good health or die early are unclear. But let's speculate. Social relationships probably influence health, either by promoting a sense of meaning and purpose in life, which enhances health, or by bringing about positive lifestyle habits in terms of sleep, nutrition, and exercise.

Let me share an example. A beloved family member did not look well at a reunion. Several of us suggested a checkup. The evaluation revealed a potentially serious situation that was remedied, and our family member should expect a full and speedy recovery. If he had been alone, the outcome might not have been so favorable.

At a family celebration, another friend of mine spotted a strange-looking mole on her brother-in-law's ear. She asked if it was new. He said it had recently appeared. He loved to cycle and was often out pedaling without sunscreen and a hat. He didn't think a thing of the dark buttonlike growth, but she suggested he have it looked at by a dermatologist. Turns out it was melanoma, and after surgery, he has a favorable outlook. Now he's a proponent of sunscreen for everyone. Had the growth gone unchecked, who knows his outcome.

Let me mention a few more scientific studies to make this point. One study looked at African-American and white women with breast cancer. Race made no difference here. But the women who had few close personal ties or people they could turn to for emotional support had an increased death rate. These findings reinforced an earlier, similar study in which stress impaired the activity of natural defensive cells among patients with breast cancer.

So what should a newly diagnosed patient with a life-threatening illness do? If he is feeling socially isolated, should he run out and try to muster all the friends he can? Does she renew old friendships at the class reunion and hope some of them stick around to shepherd her through a period of treatment and recovery?

One of the classic models of support groups has been Alcoholics Anonymous. This has been a lifesaving intervention for many men and women struggling with chemical dependency. This model has been expanded to virtually every ailment that affects humankind.

Is a support group right for you? This is a highly individual decision. As a rule of thumb, people in the chemical-dependency world have suggested that it takes attendance at four to six meetings to get a sense and a feel for the program. You can quickly decide if the group "feels right" and is good for you. You must be mindful of comparing your case to another, though, because each individual requires different management.

The verdict is still out on whether or not support systems increase length of life, but the success of these programs in most circumstances strongly suggests that the quality of life and the sense of community and connectedness cannot be ignored.

Of Hope and Guilt

Several years ago, Dr. Barri Cassileth's study was published in the *New England Journal of Medicine.* She addressed the role of attitude and disposition among the terminally ill. The paper could show no benefit of attitude whatsoever, and this resonates with another study in the *British Medical Journal,* reported in the press with this headline: "Positive mental attitude does not affect cancer survival."

How do we reconcile these findings with the general belief that attitude has something to do with illness?

An analogy might go something like this: If you are run over by a bus or a herd of buffalo, then it is highly unlikely that attitude and disposition will have anything to do with survival, because the assault on your body is completely overwhelming, and you are unable to respond. On the other hand, if you have an injury such as twisting your knee while skiing, or if you have the diagnosis of cancer and your psychological defenses are firmly rooted, then it seems logical that you may be able to marshal resources to better cope with the illness or injury. However, we need to recognize that we were genetically engineered to travel in packs and live in groups. The calf who becomes isolated from the herd has a low probability of making it to adulthood.

Remarkable patients can make the point even better:

- A Midwestern farmer had a malignant melanoma removed from his lip and had multiple spots in his lungs. He was given a dismal prognosis at his local hospital. I gave him options and alternatives, and he shared with me what these options really gave him: hope. He explained that this gave him the possibility of a reprieve. At that point, everything became crystal-clear with vibrant colors. The sky was a vivid blue. The flowers were virtually iridescent, and everything had a Technicolor, almost three-dimensional look, feel and smell. He shared with me a sense of guilt that he was spared; whereas, other good people in similar situations succumbed to their advanced cancers.

- Another middle-aged gentleman was diagnosed with an invasive, aggressive form of malignant melanoma—first spotted by his barber. The patient came to me in the middle 1980s and underwent appropriate surgery. Under the microscope this cancer had ominous characteristics and should have taken his life within a few months. That was 25 years ago. The patient has done well financially and professionally, but he has a nagging angst that he was spared for some greater good, some greater purpose, not yet clear to him.

- A prominent researcher from a well-known university is one of the foremost international academic superstars in a very narrow area of science. In the early 1980s, this researcher developed bone marrow metastasis from a malignant melanoma associated with skin lesions. The researcher received an experimental program of treatment: 19 of the

20 patients who participated in this trial died. She lived an additional 26 years. Why? The patient was accustomed to and needed the challenge of getting through the rigors of an academic environment to survive. These characteristics served her well in dealing with her disease. This is the kind of individual who would wither if abandoned on a deserted island with no sense of purpose.

- A delightful young woman developed nasal congestion. Extensive evaluations showed an angry, aggressive, high-grade cancer arising from the base of her skull. The cancer could not be removed, and it had spread to the lungs. The patient is still alive almost 30 years later. Again, a sense of connectedness and purpose—and a need to be present for her young children—were clearly factors in her survival of a situation in which others died.

- In the mid-1980s, a factory worker from a rural area came to me with abdominal pain. He underwent an exploratory procedure in which one of our premier abdominal surgeons detected a baseball-sized mass and multiple malignant satellites with the melanoma encasing the bowel. The patient underwent surgery to remove as much of the widespread cancer as possible, but it was clearly understood that a cancer was undoubtedly left behind. Again, the survival should have been no more than a few months. He likewise did well and has continued to do well for 25-plus years. Queried as to why he did well, the patient indicated, "Somehow I just knew that I would beat this thing." Naïve? No, I don't think so. More like a belief and a confidence that there was a higher power or cosmic force protecting him.

Each of these individuals provides thought-provoking insights into the resiliency of the human spirit. Psychologist Dr. Martin Seligman has extensively written about learned optimism. The optimists of life view setbacks and catastrophes as being transient, as being specific—a bankruptcy, for example—and do not extrapolate the setbacks to all life's issues. He makes a valid point that I can speak to about these patients.

When someone receives an overwhelming diagnosis, the immune system, the soul, and cognitive or higher functions simply cease to function. Some people never get over this "funk," and their depression is intertwined with an impairment of their immunity. They succumb to their illness. The optimists, somehow, have an inner spirit and inner drive to overcome adversity. This can be learned. This is not necessarily a genetically "done deal."

Now, how do we explain the phenomenon of the patient who is highly motivated, has a solid system of support and community, and has every reason to continue to live, yet he or she succumbs to the disease? What's the explanation then?

I don't think we know why this happens in some people, and this simply reflects our ignorance about the subtleties of the mind-body connection and the need for further research and studies in this area. Nevertheless, we cannot ignore the growing legion of patients who have survived far longer than anyone would have anticipated from their operative and pathology reports.

Now some tantalizing clues have been found from animal tumor experiments. When animals, whether they are rodents or primates or dogs, are given an electric shock in an experimental setting *and* the ability to control the shock to escape from the noxious environment, those animals do well. However, when the animals are exposed to relentless pressures, relentless stresses over which they have no control, the immune system clearly deteriorates. When these animals have tumors, their survival is drastically reduced.

This means that stress has something to do with the immune system—and has something to do with survival. It is perilous to read into the studies on lab animals because we of course are not rats or mice, but this may be a small piece of the puzzle. As investigations continue, we may have better probes to precisely understand the mind-body connection.

The Four Big Questions

What gives your life enduring meaning?
What is the purpose of life?
What gets you out of bed on Monday morning?
What brings you joy?

How You Can Help Someone with a Serious Illness

John Donne said, "No man is an island." What he was really saying is that we are each part of the community. We are part of a family in a general sense. In modern times, families may be blood relatives, such as brothers and sisters and mothers and fathers. However, many of us are in a family or in a community of non-blood relatives. Now what does this mean for the patient?

From the time of antiquity, we survived by living in packs or groups. Lost creatures, separated from the pack, rarely survived alone. Likewise, from ancient scriptures, we are told that the individual who falls and has no one to carry him will perish.

High drama is played out in our hospitals every day. In most circumstances, patients have family members with them. In general, the support system can be a tremendous asset.

The family can be a remarkable ally and comfort to the patient, but families can also play a negative role. Let's look at some of the things that families can do to support and encourage patients during the journey of their lifetimes:

- **Be present.** This means simply showing up. But, you may say: "I don't know what to say." "I don't know how I can help." You don't have to *do* anything. The simple act of showing up and being present and acknowledging the person's illness can work wonders for the spirit and for the soul. Ask if the patient would like you to be present when the health care team visits. Some people clutch their privacy like a child clutches a favorite teddy bear. Others wish to have another set of ears to hear what the nurses and doctors are saying. If you are asked to leave, don't make a scene; just exit quietly. If you are asked to stay, explain later what you heard from the health care team. Use simple language, don't embellish, and share with the patient your interpretations of what was said.

- **Understand that you are not the patient.** What you might wish for yourself during this time of turmoil might not be best for the patient. It is easy to be a hero when you are not in a foxhole and not on the firing line. The nauseated, pain-wracked patient with multiple sleepless nights is hardly in an ideal position to make a treatment decision, so be respectful of how that patient feels.
- **Know when it is time to show up, and know when it is time to leave.** Patients get tired. Patients are sick. Ask the patient about the best time for visits. Please understand that fighting disease or injury is an exhausting business, and trying to maintain a stiff upper lip and happy facade for visitors takes lots of energy. Don't be discouraged or offended if patients don't want to be involved in the usual chatter about the football season, the weather, and the current race for mayor. These discussions become insignificant when faced with the 11th hour of illness. The focus is on the patient, not on you or other visitors.
- **Ask the patient what you can bring him or her.** A favorite magazine. A favorite book or video can be far more important medicine than the kind that comes in pill form. Don't ever forget the power and the energy from a card, a thoughtful e-mail, a bouquet of flowers, or a tray of homemade lasagna. A box of cookies lines the stomach and warms the soul.
- **Be there for the long term.** Make certain that the patient understands that you will be there whether the news is good or bad. As the journey unfolds, well-wishers quietly disappear. Sometimes, when the patient is most in need of support, the cast of thousands dwindles to a small number. Be among those who are counted when the going gets tough.

My Survival Rx

I have had the privilege of interacting with thousands of patients during my medical career, and some are particularly memorable. Although all are courageous, some are particularly courageous.

You met Chris in the foreword of this book. I first met this young man in the early 1990s. He had positive lymph nodes being replaced by malignant melanoma under his armpit. The probability of survival then was zero. He returned to see me at three-month intervals initially, now every six months, and remains well today. His family, especially his children, are undoubtedly factors in his survival.

Twenty years ago, there were no proven therapies for Chris's situation, and the experimental treatments were not promising. After thoughtful discussions with him and his family, we all agreed that proactive, aggressive surveillance, with a careful history and physical exam and appropriate scans every several months, would be reasonable. Today, he continues to see me. He's an established professional in his career. What is the lesson?

I do not have all the answers, but I can tell you that attitude, disposition, and a supportive environment have something to do with surviving cancer or any life-threatening illness. We all recognize that some studies do not show the impact of attitude and disposition, but we cannot ignore these remarkable patients who defy the odds and somehow live meaningful, productive, and creative lives in the face of a devastating prognosis. Chris and others defy the odds, rewrite the books, and provide hope and inspiration for us all.

Also at play here were early diagnoses, careful decision making about treatment, a savvy patient willing to make important lifestyle changes, a supportive family, a superb doctor-patient relationship—all key to navigating a changing medical system, to living a healthy life, and to surviving any diagnosis, which is my message to you in this book.

Thank you for reading. I now urge you to make meaningful lifestyle changes and to be vigilant about your health ... so you will not be my patient.

References and Resources

The authors have cited scientific studies and reports. The following are citations and web addresses for readers who wish to view the original sources for this book when first published in 2003 and extensively updated in 2014. As always, web addresses often change. These were current as of this printing.

Chapter 1: The Race Against Time

AARP. "Beyond 50: A Report to the Nation on Trends in Health Security." May 21, 2002.

Barzilai, Nir, and colleagues. "Lifestyle Factors of People with Exceptional Longevity." *Journal of the American Geriatrics Society* (July 28, 2011).

Blendon, R. J., and colleagues. "Americans' Health Priorities: Curing Cancer and Controlling Costs." *Health Affairs* 20 (November/December 2001): 222–32.

Creagan, E. T. "The Disease Americans Fear Most, Why They Don't Have To." Health-eheadlines Consumer Health News Service (*health-eheadlines.com*), 2012.

He, Wan, and Mark N. Muenchrath. "90+ in the United States: 2006–2008." National Institutes of Health, November 17, 2011.

MetLife Foundation. "What America Thinks." MetLife Foundation Alzheimer's Survey (*metlife.com*), February 2011.

Moynihan, R. I., and colleagues. "Selling Sickness: The Pharmaceutical Industry and Disease Mongering." *British Medical Journal* 324 (April 13, 2002): 886–91.

Oeppen, J., and J. W. Vaupel. "Demography. Broken Limits to Life Expectancy." *Science* 296 (May 10, 2002): 1029–31.

Scott, Joy. "The Impact of the Baby Boomers on Healthcare Marketing." *HealthLeaders.com*, May 8, 2002.

Society for Women's Health Research, Fact Sheet (*womens-health.org*).

Chapter 2: Pack Your Own Parachute

Barzilai, D. A., and colleagues. "Does Health Habit Counseling Affect Patient Satisfaction?" *American Journal of Preventive Medicine* 33 (October 24, 2001): 595–99.

Dubbert, P. M. "Physical Activity and Exercise: Recent Advances and Current Challenges." *Journal of Consulting and Clinical Psychology* 70 (2002): 526–36.

Prochaska, J. O., John C. Norcross, and Carlos Diclemente. *Changing for Good*. New York: Avon Books, 1995.

Chapter 3: How to Talk So Your Doctor Will Listen

Bell, R. A, and colleagues. "Unsaid But Not Forgotten: Patients' Unvoiced Desires in Office Visits." *Archives of Internal Medicine* 161 (September 10, 2001): 1977–84.

Deyo, R. A. "A Key Medical Decision Maker: The Patient." *British Medical Journal* 323 (September 1, 2001): 466–7.

Epstein, R. H. "Major Medical Mystery: Why People Avoid Doctors." *The New York Times*, October 31, 2000.

Friedberg, M. K., and colleagues. "Factors Affecting Physician Professional Satisfaction and Their Implications for Patient Care, Health Systems, and Health Policy." RAND Health (*rand.org*), 2013.

Geraghty, E. M., and colleagues. "Primary Care Visit Length, Quality, and Satisfaction for Standardized Patients with Depression." *Journal of General Internal Medicine* 22 (December 2007): 1641–47.

Gottschalk, A., and S. A. Flocke. "Time Spent in Face-to-Face Patient Care and Work Outside the Examination Room." *Annals of Family Medicine* 3 (November 2005): 488–93.

King, K., and H. T. Reis. "Marriage and Long-Term Survival After Coronary Artery Bypass Grafting." *Health Psychology* 31 (January 2012): 55–62.

Langewitz, W., and colleagues. "Spontaneous Talking Time at Start of Consultation in Outpatient Clinic: Cohort Study." *British Medical Journal* 325 (September 28, 2002): 682–3.

Mayo Clinic. "Five Ways Patients and Care Providers Can Improve Health Care." Press release, Mayo Clinic newsroom, June 11, 2013.

Mechanic, D., and colleagues. "Are Patients' Office Visits with Physicians Getting Shorter?" *New England Journal of Medicine* 344 (January 18, 2001): 198–204.

Montague, E., and colleagues. "Nonverbal Interpersonal Interactions in Clinical Encounters and Patient Perceptions of Empathy." *Journal of Participatory Medicine* 5 (August 14, 2013): n.p.

National Center for Health Statistics. "Health, United States, 2012." 2013.

Pew Internet & American Life. "Vital Decisions: How Internet Users Decide What Information to Trust When They or Their Loved Ones Are Sick." May 22, 2002.

Rhoades, D. R., and colleagues. "Speaking and Interruptions During Primary Care Office Visits." *Family Medicine* 33 (July/August 2001): 528–32.

Roter, D. L., and colleagues. "Physician Gender Effects in Medical Communication: A Meta-Analytic Review." *Journal of the American Medical Association* (*JAMA*) 288 (August 14, 2002): 756–64.

Schiller, J. S., and colleagues. "Summary Health Statistics for U.S. Adults: National Health Interview Survey, 2011." Centers for Disease Control and Prevention (CDC), Division of Health Interview Statistics, December 2012.

Whitlock, E. P., and colleagues. "Evaluating Primary Care Behavioral Counseling Interventions: An Evidence-based Approach." *American Journal of Preventive Medicine* 22 (May 2002): 267–84.

Chapter 4: What They Never Taught Me in Medical School

Cooper, R. A., and colleagues. "Economic and Demographic Trends Signal an Impending Physician Shortage." *Health Affairs* 21 (January/February 2002): 140–54.

Creagan, E. T. "Bombarded by Stress. Healthy Habits to Avert Burnout." *Minnesota Medicine* 82 (August 1999): 14–5, 49.

Creagan, E. T. "Stress among Medical Oncologists: The Phenomenon of Burnout and a Call to Action." *Mayo Clinic Proceedings* 68 (June 1993): 614–5.

Inlander, C. "Warning: Your Hospital Can Make You Sick: How to Protect Yourself." *Bottom Line/Personal*, April 1, 2002.

Morrison, I. "The Future of Physician's Time." *Annals of Internal Medicine* 132 (January 4, 2000): 80–4.

"Physician Burnout: Packing Your Career Survival Kit" (interview with Edward T. Creagan, M.D.). *Mayo Alumni*, Fall/Winter 1997.

Rennard, B. O., and colleagues. "Chicken Soup Inhibits Neutrophil Chemotaxis in Vitro." *Chest* 118 (October 2000): 1150–7.

Chapter 5: How to Be an Empowered Patient

Institute of Medicine. "To Err Is Human: Building a Safer Health System." 1999.

James, J. T. "A New, Evidence-Based Estimate of Patient Harms Associated with Hospital Care." *Journal of Patient Safety* 9 (September 2013): 122–28.

Chapter 6: What Should I Get Screened For?

Centers for Disease Control and Prevention (CDC). "Recommended Adult Immunization Schedule—United States, 2013" (*cdc.gov*).

Etzioni, R., and colleagues. "Overdiagnosis Due to Prostate Specific Antigen Screening: Lessons from U.S. Prostate Cancer Incidence Trends." *Journal of the National Cancer Institute* 94 (July 13, 2002): 981–90.

Harris, R., and K. N. Lohr. "Screening for Prostate Cancer: An Update of the Evidence for the U.S. Preventive Services Task Force." *Annals of Internal Medicine* 137 (December 3, 2002): 917–29.

Jaramillo, E., and colleagues. "Variation Among Primary Care Physicians in Prostate-Specific Antigen Screening of Older Men." *JAMA* 310 (2013): 1622–24.

Laine C. "The Annual Physical Examination: Needless Ritual or Necessary Routine?" *Annals of Internal Medicine* 136 (May 7, 2002): 701–3.

Landers, S. J. "Full-Body Scans: Buying Peace of Mind." *amednews.com,* September 3, 2001.

Squiers, L. B., and colleagues. "Prostate-Specific Antigen Testing: Men's Responses to the 2012 Recommendations Against Screening." *American Journal of Preventive Medicine* 45 (2013): 182–189.

Chapter 7: Your Prevention Prescription

American Academy of Allergy, Asthma and Immunology and the Environmental Protection Agency. Smoke Free Home Pledge Campaign (*aaaai.org*).

American Academy of Dermatology. A 2.5-minute video from the American Academy of Dermatology demonstrates how to check your skin for suspicious moles and what to look for. Search on YouTube.com.

American Cancer Society. Facts About Secondhand Smoke and Restaurants (*cancer.org*).

American College of Sports Medicine. "ACSM's Guidelines for Exercise Testing" (*acsm.org*).

Axmaker, Larry. *Real Men Get Prostate Cancer Too: The Information You Want Your Doctor to Tell You But You're Too Scared to Ask* (second edition). Molalla, Oregon: Olde & Graye Publishing, 2012.

Barkley, J., and A. Lepp. "Professors Connect Cell Phone Use with Inactivity." Press release. Kent State University, July 16, 2013.

Berk, L. S., and colleagues. "Neuroendocrine and Stress Hormone Changes During Mirthful Laughter." *American Journal of the Medical Sciences* 298 (December 1989): 390–6.

Berk, L. S., and colleagues. "Modulation of Neuro-Immune Parameters During the Eustress of Humor-Associated Mirthful Laughter." *Alternative Therapies in Health and Medicine* 7 (March 2001): 62–76.

Berk, L. S., and colleagues. "Laughercise: Health Benefits Similar to Exercise Lowers Cholesterol and Systolic Blood Pressure." Association of Psychological Science, San Francisco, May 2009.

Berk, L. S., and colleagues. "Mirthful Laughter as Adjunct Therapy in Diabetic Care, Increases HDL Cholesterol and Attenuates Inflammatory Cytokines and hs-CRP." FASEB Experimental Biology, American Physiological Society, April 2009.

Bishop, T., and colleagues. "Electronic Communication Improves Access, But Barriers to Its Widespread Adoption Remain." *Health Affairs* 32 (August 2013): 81361–7.

Blackburn, E. "What Do Mothers of Children with Special Needs and Combat Soldiers Have in Common? STRESS" *(abilitypath.org)*.

Breslow, L., and N. Breslow. "Health Practices and Disability: Some Evidence from Alameda County." *American Journal of Preventive Medicine* 22 (January 1993): 86–95.

Bureau of Labor Statistics. "American Time Use Survey." 2011.

Calorie Control Council. "Most Americans Are Weight Conscious." Press release, April 27, 2011 *(caloriecontrol.org)*.

Centers for Disease Control and Prevention (CDC). "Insufficient Sleep Is a Public Health Epidemic." March 14, 2013 *(cdc.gov/features/dssleep)*.

Centers for Disease Control and Prevention (CDC). "One in Five Adults Meets Overall Physical Activity Guidelines." *Morbidity and Mortality Weekly Report,* May 2, 2013.

Centers for Disease Control and Prevention (CDC). "Obesity and Overweight" *(cdc.gov/nchs/fastats/overwt.htm)*.

Centers for Disease Control and Prevention (CDC). "Overweight and Obesity" (*cdc.gov/obesity/data/adult.html*).

Centers for Disease Control and Prevention (CDC). "Smoking & Tobacco Use" (*cdc.gov/tobacco/data_statistics/fact_sheets/fast_facts/*).

Creagan, E. T. "Malignant Melanoma: An Emerging and Preventable Medical Catastrophe." *Mayo Clinic Proceedings* 72 (June 1997): 570–4.

Crichton, G. E., and colleagues. "Relation Between Dairy Food Intake and Cognitive Function: The Maine-Syracuse Longitudinal Study." *International Dairy Journal* 22 (2012): 15–23.

EHSToday. Infographic: Four Distracted Driving Myths (*ehstoday.com/print/safety/infographic-four-distracted-driving-myths*).

Eliot, R. S. *From Stress to Strength: How to Lighten Your Load and Save Your Life*. New York: Bantam, 1994.

Eliot, R. S., and D. L. Breo. *Is It Worth Dying For? A Self-Assessment Program to Make Stress Work for You, Not Against You*. New York: Bantam Doubleday, 1991.

Food and Drug Administration (FDA). E-Cigarettes: Questions and Answers. September 2010 (*fda.gov/ForConsumers/ConsumerUpdates/ucm225210.htm*).

Grandey, A. A. "Emotion Regulation in the Workplace: A New Way to Conceptualize Emotional Labor." *Journal of Occupational Health Psychology* 5 (January 2000): 95–110.

Greer, S., and colleagues. "The Impact of Sleep Deprivation on Food Desire in the Human Brain," *Nature Communications,* August 2013.

Harris Interactive. "Tech Stress: How Many E-mails Can You Handle a Day?" July 20, 2010.

Holford, T. and colleagues. "Tobacco Control and the Reduction in Smoking-Related Premature Deaths in the United States, 1964–2012." *JAMA* 311 (January 2014): 164–171.

Institute of Medicine, National Academy of Sciences. "Dietary Reference Intakes for Energy, Carbohydrate, Fiber, Fat, Fatty Acids, Cholesterol, Protein, and Amino Acids (Macronutrients)." September 2002 (*iom.edu*).

Jacobs, T. L., and colleagues. "Intensive Meditation Training, Immune Cell Telomerase Activity, and Psychological Mediators." *Psychoneuroendocrinology* 36 (June 2011): 664–81.

Jeans, E. A., and colleagues. "Translation of Exercise Testing to Exercise Prescription Using the Talk Test." *Journal of Strength & Conditioning Research* 25 (March 2011): 590–96.

Kobuszewski, A. *Food: Field to Fork, How to Grow Sustainably, Shop Wisely, Cook Nutritiously, and Eat Deliciously.* AnitaBeHealthy, 2011.

Maruta, T., and colleagues. "Optimism-Pessimism Assessed in the 1960s and Self-Reported Health Status 30 Years Later." *Mayo Clinic Proceedings* 77 (August 2002): 748–53.

Miller, A. and colleagues. "Twenty-five Year Follow-up for Breast Cancer Incidence and Mortality of the Canadian National Breast Screening Study: Randomised Screening Trial." *British Medical Journal* 348 (January 2014): 366.

National Highway Traffic Safety Administration. Drowsy Driving and Automobile Crashes (*nhlbi.nih.gov/health/prof/sleep/drsy_drv.pdf*).

National Institute on Aging. Exercise: A Guide from the National Institute of Aging (*nih.gov/nia*).

National Sleep Foundation. "Sleep in America" survey. 2013.

Nelson, M. E., and colleagues. "Effects of High-Intensity Strength Training on Multiple Risk Factors for Osteoporotic Fractures. A Randomized Controlled Trial. *JAMA* 272 (December 28, 1994): 1909–14.

Nelson, M., and J. Ackerman. *The Social Network Diet: Change Yourself, Change the World.* FastPencil, 2011.

Pew Research, Religion & Public Life Project. "Living to 120 and Beyond: Americans' Views on Aging, Medical Advances and Radical Life Extension." August 6, 2013.

Physician Wellness Services and Cejka Search. "Study from Physician Wellness Services and Cejka Search Reveals Nearly 87 Percent of Physicians are Moderately to Severely Stressed." Press release, *BusinessWire,* November 29, 2011.

President's Council on Fitness, Sports & Nutrition. "Physical Activity Guidelines for Americans." 2008. (*fitness.gov*).

Puterman, E., and colleagues. "The Power of Exercise: Buffering the Effect of Chronic Stress on Telomere Length." *PLoS One* 5 (May 2010).

Quinn, C., and colleagues. "Type 2 Diabetes Mobile App." *Diabetes Care*, September 2011.

Rolls, B.J. "The Role of Energy Density in the Overconsumption of Fat." *Journal of Nutrition* 130 (February 2000): 268S–271S.

Rolls, B.J., and colleagues. "Portion Size of Food Affects Energy Intake in Normal-Weight and Overweight Men and Women." *American Journal of Clinical Nutrition* (December 2002): 1207–13.

Sacks, F. M., and colleagues. "Effects on Blood Pressure of Reduced Dietary Sodium and the Dietary Approaches to Stop Hypertension (DASH) Diet. DASH-Sodium Collaborative Research Group." *New England Journal of Medicine* 344 (January 2001): 3–10.

Sands, W. A., and J. R. McNeal. "A Kinematic Comparison of Four Abdominal Training Devices and a Traditional Abdominal Crunch." *Journal of Strength and Conditioning Research* 16 (February 2002): 135–41.

Warber, S., and colleagues. "Healing the Heart: A Randomized Pilot Study of a Spiritual Retreat for Depression in Acute Coronary Syndrome Patients." *Explore: the Journal of Science and Healing* (July 2011).

Wendel, S. "The Secret of Life." In LiveWell special supplement, *Omaha World-Herald,* 2011.

Chapter 9: The Search for Health, Peace, and Serenity in Complementary Medicine

Becker, M., and D. Morton. *The Healing Power of Pets.* New York: Hyperion, 2002.

Benson, H. *The Relaxation Response.* New York: Avon, 1990.

Benson, H., and W. Proctor. *Beyond the Relaxation Response: How to Harness the Healing Power of Your Personal Beliefs.* New York: Berkley, 1994.

Benson, H., and colleagues. "Study of the Therapeutic Effects of Intercessory Prayer (STEP) in Cardiac Bypass Patients: A Multicenter Randomized Trial of Uncertainty and Certainty of Receiving Intercessory Prayer." *American Heart Journal* 151 (April 2006): 934–42.

Bernardi, L., and colleagues. "Effect of Rosary Prayer and Yoga Mantras on Autonomic Cardiovascular Rhythms: Comparative Study." *British Medical Journal* 323 (December 22–29, 2001): 1446–9.

Clair, A. A. "The Effects of Music Therapy on Engagement in Family Caregiver and Care Receiver Couples with Dementia." *American Journal of Alzheimer's Disease and Other Dementias* 17 (September/ October 2002): 286–90.

Cousins, N. *Anatomy of an Illness as Perceived by the Patient: Reflections on Healing and Regeneration.* New York: Bantam Doubleday, 1991.

Deljanin Ilic, M., and colleagues. "Do Patients with Heart Failure Have Equal Response of Endothelial Function as Patients Without Heart Failure to Exercise Training?" European Society of Cardiology, ESC Congress, 2013.

Kessler, R. C., and colleagues. "The Use of Complementary and Alternative Therapies to Treat Anxiety and Depression in the United States." *American Journal of Psychiatry* 158 (February 2001): 289–94.

Kessler, R. C., and colleagues. "Long-Term Trends in the Use of Complementary and Alternative Medical Therapies in the United States." *Annals of Internal Medicine* 135 (August 2001): 262–8.

Levine, G. N., and colleagues. "Pet Ownership and Cardiovascular Risk: A Scientific Statement from the American Heart Association." *Circulation*, online, May 9, 2013.

Mayo Clinic, Edward T. Creagan blog. "Pets and Your Health: The Power of Puppy Love."

McConnell, A. R., and colleagues. "Friends with Benefits: On the Positive Consequences of Pet Ownership." *Journal of Personality and Social Psychology*, online, July 4, 2011.

Moertel, C. G., and colleagues. "A Clinical Trial of Amygdalin (Laetrile) in the Treatment of Human Cancer." *New England Journal of Medicine* 306 (January 1982): 201–6.

Moertel, C. G., and colleagues (including author E. T. Creagan). "High-Dose Vitamin C Versus Placebo in the Treatment of Patients with Advanced Cancer Who Have Had No Prior Chemotherapy. A Randomized Double-Blind Comparison." *New England Journal of Medicine* 312 (January 1985): 137–41.

National Institutes of Health, National Center for Complementary and Alternative Medicine. "What Is Complementary and Alternative Medicine (CAM)?" (*nccam.nih.gov*).

Chapter 10: Attitude Matters: The Psychology of Survival and Longevity

Allen, K., and colleagues. "Cardiovascular Reactivity and the Presence of Pets, Friends, and Spouses: The Truth About Cats and Dogs." *Psychosomatic Medicine* 64 (September/October 2002): 727–39.

Bretscher, M. E., and E. T. Creagan. "Understanding Suffering: What Palliative Medicine Teaches Us." *Mayo Clinic Proceedings* 72 (August 1997): 785–7.

Byock, Ira. *The Best Care Possible: A Physician's Quest to Transform Care Through the End of Life*. New York: Avery, 2012.

Cassileth, B. R., and colleagues. "Survival and Quality of Life Among Patients Receiving Unproven as Compared with Conventional Cancer Therapy." *New England Journal of Medicine* 324 (April 1991): 1180–5.

Creagan, E. T. "How to Break Bad News and Not Devastate the Patient." *Mayo Clinic Proceedings* 69 (October 1994): 1015–7.

Creagan, E. T. "Attitude and Disposition: Do They Make a Difference in Cancer Survival?" *Mayo Clinic Proceedings* 72 (February 1997): 160–4.

Krucoff, M. W., and colleagues. "Integrative Noetic Therapies as Adjuncts to Percutaneous Intervention during Unstable Coronary Syndromes: Monitoring and Actualization of Noetic Training (MANTRA) Feasibility Pilot." *American Heart Journal* 152 (November 2001): 760–9.

Maruta, T., and colleagues. "Optimism-Pessimism Assessed in the 1960s and Self-Reported Health Status 30 Years Later." *Mayo Clinic Proceedings* 77 (August 2002): 748–53.

Strawbridge, W. J., and colleagues. "Religious Attendance Increases Survival by Improving and Maintaining Good Health Behaviors, Mental Health, and Social Relationships." *Annals of Behavioral Medicine* 23 (Winter 2001): 68–74.

Acknowledgments

The secret of longevity is community. We need people, we need community, and we need support to go the distance. This is true in life. This is true in creating a book. Let me thank my community.

First, I thank, and dedicate this book to, the thousands of patients and their families whom I have had the privilege of knowing over a 37-year career. Each is a hero, each is a heroine, and each has pushed on in the face of numbing odds and incredible challenges that would wither the spirit of the most professional performer. I have marveled at how they have held their lives together in the face of a relentless disease called cancer.

To my Mayo Clinic and Rochester, Minnesota, team: Monica Sveen-Ziebell of Medical Relations, who helped guide the administrative process; attorney Mark Utz; colleague Dr. Scott Litin; medical transcriptionists Patti Chiarini in Rochester and Shari Hendrick in Omaha, who know it takes this village and more.

My wife, my best friend, Peggy Menzel, has been with me on each step of the journey. Without her support, encouragement, and critical eye, none of this would have been possible. My three adult sons, Ed, Matt, and Adam, are out on their own but were strong supports from day 1.

Physicians owe their careers to many individuals who guided them. To my professors, my mentors, my colleagues, I can only say, thank you for the privilege of your support and your encouragement.

The first professional colleague to review the initial manuscript was Dr. Leonard Gunderson, one of the foremost radiation oncologists in the world. Dr. Gunderson was the chair of our

Department of Oncology at Mayo Clinic. I thank him for his insight and counsel.

This effort also benefited immeasurably from the relentless review and wise guidance of Dr. Robert Dalton from the Mayo Clinic Health System. And a wag of the tail to Dr. Marty Becker, one of our nation's most beloved veterinarians and experts on the healing power of pets.

We have been blessed with a marvelous production and marketing team: Lou Anne Baker of LADESIGNCO for a winning cover design; Steven and Joe of Mudd Hill Movies for a powerful book promo; Bob Vaaler and his genius behind a video camera; Concierge Marketing, Inc., in Omaha, with sincere thanks for the wise advice of Lisa Pelto; an unmatched editorial team, including Lisa Drucker, the editor who tirelessly reviewed every word, every semicolon, every comma, with devoted attention to the healing power of the written word in a book such as this.

Now let me turn to the one person who has been the catalyst, the flame, the engine driving this project: Sandra Wendel. My tenacious and patient collaborator is the consummate wordsmith who magically transformed our ideas from a casual telephone conversation several years ago into a masterpiece—again.

And to all the readers of the first edition who have thanked me in person and by phone or e-mail over the years—and all those who may do so as our journey unfolds—thank you for being empowered patients and caregivers. You are my raison d'être.

INDEX

About the Author

Edward T. Creagan, M.D., F.A.A.H.P.M., is a professor of medical oncology at the Mayo Clinic Medical School. He holds the endowed chair as the John and Roma Rouse Professor of Humanism in Medicine. Most recently, he was named Outstanding Educator from the Mayo Clinic School of Continuing Medical Education and has received the Distinguished Mayo Clinician Award—Mayo Clinic's highest honor. He completed an elected term as President of the Mayo Staff.

Dr. Creagan was the first Mayo Clinic consultant board certified in hospice and palliative medicine. He is a Fellow of the American Academy of Hospice and Palliative Medicine.

Dr. Creagan received his medical training at New York Medical College and earned graduate degrees in internal medicine and oncology at the University of Michigan and the National Cancer Institute before joining the staff at the Mayo Clinic in Rochester, Minnesota, where he has endured over 37 Minnesota winters. He is board certified in internal medicine, medical oncology, and hospice medicine and palliative care.

He is the author of over 400 scientific papers and has given 1,000 presentations throughout the world, including his home state of New Jersey. His columns on health, wellness, and the mind-body connection have appeared in Midwestern newspapers. He tweets @EdwardCreagan and @AskDoctorEd and blogs on *MayoClinic.com,* Mayo Clinic's online website for consumer health information, where

Dr. Creagan is associate medical editor. He is the editor of the book *Mayo Clinic on Healthy Aging.*

An avid marathoner and golfer, father of three sons, grandfather of two incredible boys, Dr. Creagan and his wife, Peggy, live in Rochester, Minnesota.

Collaborator **Sandra Wendel** is an Omaha-based journalist and consumer health-information writer. Her stories appear on the top health websites, including her own Health-eheadlines Consumer Health News Service (*health-eheadlines.com*). She has contributed to *eMedicineHealth.com* and *MayoClinic.com*. She is a regular contributor to *LiveWell*, the health section for the *Omaha World-Herald*, writes a column called Be Well for the *Inspired Living Omaha* magazine, and writes environmental features for the farm-to-fork magazine *Edible Omaha*. She is an independent book editor and publishing consultant, a journalism graduate of the University of Iowa, and instructor of book writing and publishing at Metropolitan Community College. Contact Sandra through *SandraWendel.com*.

Contact the Author: Please understand that Dr. Creagan cannot diagnose or review your personal medical information, but he welcomes your feedback and comments through the website for this book at *HowNotToBeMyPatient.com*.